A Clinician's Guide to ADHD

Joseph Sadek

A Clinician's Guide to ADHD

Second Edition

Springer

Joseph Sadek
Department of Psychiatry
Dalhousie University
Halifax
Nova Scotia
Canada

The work was first published in 2013 by Dr. Joseph Sadek as online publication

ISBN 978-3-319-02358-8 ISBN 978-3-319-02359-5 (eBook)
DOI 10.1007/978-3-319-02359-5
Springer Cham Heidelberg New York Dordrecht London

Library of Congress Control Number: 2013954597

Printed on acid-free paper

Springer is part of Springer Science+Business Media (www.springer.com)

I want to give my sincere thanks and gratitude to my wife Irene and my children Joseph and Maryanne who were extremely supportive during the journey of producing this book.
I would also like to express my sincere appreciation and gratitude to my fellow board members, and to the staff, of CADDRA for their continued support.

Disclaimer

The text in this book, and its references, are for education, guidance, and information purposes only. Responsibility remains in hands of the clinician diagnosing and treating their own patient to determine the correct course for their patient. No one who took part in creating this text can be held legally responsible for any of the -information contained in the text.

Foreword

Attention deficit hyperactivity disorder (ADHD) is a medical condition arising from perturbations in brain functioning that lead to an individual showing challenges in sustained attention, excessive non-goal directed motor activity and enhanced impulsivity. These result in significant and substantial long and short term problems in daily life, including: social and interpersonal difficulties; poorer academic and vocational achievement and a much higher risk for negative life outcomes such as traffic accidents, drug abuse, marital discord and job losses. Like in any medical condition, these challenges play themselves out in complex social circumstances. Also, as in many medical conditions, ADHD is treatable. And, with the right treatments, provided over the necessary period of time, most people who have ADHD can recover and do well.

The challenges that health providers have had in dealing with ADHD include: trying to ensure that the best science is used to help in the diagnosis and treatment of those who have ADHD, that those who require treatment receive it and that those who receive treatment get the most appropriate interventions to meet their unique needs. This can be a difficult challenge, because life is different for every person who has ADHD and thus treatment for each person needs to be provided in a manner that is both directed by the scientific evidence and based on their personal needs and strengths.

Dr. Joseph Sadek has, in this book, taken an important step in providing information and understanding that can help health providers better diagnose and treat those who live with ADHD. He has done this by bringing together available and current scientific evidence and has melded this with important and clinically useful considerations for care. And, he has done so in a manner that is easily accessible for the busy health provider and the informed reader alike.

This new resource can go a long way in helping improve the lives of people who live with ADHD.

Dalhousie University Stan Kutcher

Copyrights/Permissions

Contents

1 Introduction

There is a need for a clear and concise approach to a complex disorder such as Attention Deficit Hyperactivity Disorder (ADHD). This guide combines the useful approaches used in different guidelines with the recent literature reviews, clinical expertise, and other web resources.

The approach to gathering information from guidelines was broad. Guidelines were collected from different REGIONS such as North America (CADDRA for Canadian guidelines, and ACAP and others for American guidelines), Australia (Australian draft guidelines), and Europe (NICE, British, Scottish and others).

This guide is intended for educational purposes only. There are different areas in the field of ADHD that were not captured in this guide and readers are encouraged to continue to update their knowledge regularly.

J. Sadek, *A Clinician's Guide to ADHD*,
DOI 10.1007/978-3-319-02359-5_1,

History of Attention Deficit Hyperactivity Disorder

2

2.1 Early History of ADHD

Contributors to ADHD development have been numerous over a surprising period of time. Here is a brief overview of some of the early history of ADHD as reported by some authors:

Sir Alexander Crichton

The first example of a disorder that appears to be similar to ADHD was given by a Scottish physician Sir Alexander Crichton in 1798. In his publication, "An inquiry into the nature and origin of mental derangement", he mentioned "the incapacity of attending with a necessary degree of constancy to any one object". According to Crichton, the incapacity of attending, if not innate, can also be caused by nervous disorders. This notion was later rediscovered in the concepts of minimal brain damage or dysfunction. His work came after the German physician Melchior Adam Weikard who published a medical text book in 1775 which included a chapter called Attention Disorders.

Heinrich Hoffmann

In 1844, the German physician Heinrich Hoffmann created some illustrated children's stories including "Fidgety Phil". The description fits the hyperactive type of ADHD very well.

Sir George Frederic Still

The lectures of Sir George Frederic Still in 1902 are considered by many well-known authors, such as Barkley and Conners, to be the scientific starting point of the history of ADHD. Still described 20 cases of children with a "defect of moral control as a morbid manifestation, without general impairment of intellect and without physical disease".

Alfred Frank Tredgold

Tredgold in 1908 discussed a correlation between early brain damage, for example, caused by birth defect or perinatal anoxia, and subsequent behavior problems or learning difficulties. At that time, epidemic encephalitis was spreading around the world; the residual effect of the encephalitis had many similarities to several ADHD symptoms. The concept of Post Encephalitic Behavior disorder was

J. Sadek, *A Clinician's Guide to ADHD*,
DOI 10.1007/978-3-319-02359-5_2, © Springer International Publishing Switzerland 2014

introduced then. Also, Tredgold was the first to discuss the importance of modifying the environment as part of the management of this disorder.

Franz Kramer and Hans Pollnow

In 1932, the German physicians Franz Kramer and Hans Pollnow reported on a hyperkinetic disease of infancy "the most characteristic symptom of affected children was a marked motor restlessness. The children are described as unable to stay still for a second, climb about preferring high furniture in particular." They also described several other features of ADHD.

Charles Bradley

In 1937, Charles Bradley from Rhode Island reported a positive effect of stimulant medication in children with various behavior disorders. This was the first description of the effect of stimulant treatment on ADHD. He used racemic amphetamine product.

Leandro Panizzon

Methylphenidate was first synthesized in 1944 by Leandro Panizzon and marketed as "Ritalin" by Ciba-Geigy Pharmaceutical Company in 1954. The name "Ritalin" derives from the first name of Panizzon's wife, i.e. Marguerite or "Rita".

2.2 The Next Evolution of Discoveries in ADHD

2.2.1 Minimal Brain Damage and Minimal Brain Dysfunction

The concept of minimal brain damage was popular particularly between 1930 and 1940. Many authors concluded that hyperactivity in children may be caused by damage to the brain. The new concept of "minimal brain damage" was based on several considerations. First, Tredgold had stated that mild forms of brain damage in infancy, although unnoticed at the time, could lead to behavioral sequelae which first became apparent at school (Ross and Ross 1976). Second, possible variations of brain damage extent, locus, or type of lesion were discussed. Third, the concept of "a continuum of cerebral damage ranging from severe abnormalities, such as cerebral palsy and mental deficiency, to minimal damage" was introduced by Knobloch and Pasamanick in 1959.

Despite the fact this hypothesis stated that a minimal brain damage may lead to behavior disorders was well established and popular, many challenged the concept, particularly in 1960. Some researchers found children with hyperkinetic impulse without the classic etiologic traumatic or infectious factors in their history. They suggested a functional disturbance, rather than damage to the brain, as the cause of the characteristic syndrome. In 1963, the Oxford International Study Group of Child Neurology (Bax and MacKeith 1963) held a conference and stated that brain damage should not be inferred from problematic behavior signs alone. They advocated a shift in terminology by replacing the term "minimal brain damage" with "minimal brain dysfunction".

2.2.2 Historical Review of DSM Definition of ADHD

(DSM-II 1968)

The second edition of the Diagnostic and Statistical Manual of Mental Disorders (DSM-II) mentioned "Hyperkinetic Reaction of Childhood" and defined it two sentences: "The disorder is characterized by over activity, restlessness, distractibility, and short attention span, especially in young children; the behavior usually diminishes by adolescence" (American Psychiatric Association 1968).

(DSM-III 1980)

The third edition of the Diagnostic and Statistical Manual of Mental Disorders (DSM-III) mentioned Attention Deficit Disorder: with and without hyperactivity. In 1987 with DSM-III-R, the concept of two subtypes was removed and renamed the "Attention Deficit-Hyperactivity Disorder (ADHD) disorder." The symptoms of inattention, impulsivity, and hyperactivity were combined into a single list of symptoms with a single cutoff score (American Psychiatric Association 1980).

(DSM-IV 1994)

ADHD was subdivided into three subtypes, i.e. a predominantly inattentive type, a predominantly hyperactive-impulsive type, and a combined type with symptoms of both dimensions (American Psychiatric Association 1994).

References and Recommended Readings

American Psychiatric Association (ed) (1987) Diagnostic and statistical manual of mental disorders: DSM-III-TR®. American Psychiatric Pub

American Psychiatric Association (ed) (1968) Diagnostic and statistical manual of mental disorders: DSM-II®. American Psychiatric Pub, Washington, DC

American Psychiatric Association (ed) (1980) Diagnostic and statistical manual of mental disorders: DSM-III®. American Psychiatric Pub, Washington, DC

American Psychiatric Association (ed) (1994) Diagnostic and statistical manual of mental disorders: DSM-IV®. American Psychiatric Pub, Washington, DC

Barkley RA, Peters H (2012) The earliest reference to ADHD in the medical literature? Melchior Adam Weikard's description in 1775 of "attention deficit" (mangel der aufmerksamkeit, attentio volubilis). J Attent Disord 16(8):623–630

Bax M, MacKeith R, International study group at Oxford (1963) Minimal cerebral dysfunction. Clin Dev Med 10:1–20

Crichton A (1798) An inquiry into the nature and origin of mental derangement. Cadell & Davies, London

Lange KW, Reichl S, Lange KM, Tucha L, Tucha O (2010) The history of attention deficit hyperactivity disorder. Atten Defic Hyperact Disord 2(4):241–255

Pasamanick B, Knobloch H (1960) Brain and behavior. Symposium, 1959. 2. Brain damage and reproductive casualty. Am J Orthopsychiatry 30:298

Ross DM, Ross Sa (1976) Hyperactivity: research theory and action. New York, Wiley

Taylor E (2011) Antecedents of ADHD: a historical account of diagnostic concepts. Atten Defic Hyperact Disord 3(2):69–75

3 Epidemiology and Etiology of ADHD

3.1 Epidemiology

ADHD is the most common psychiatric disorder of childhood. Overall, prevalence ranges from 5 to 12 % in school-aged children. Male to female ratio is around 3:1 in children and adolescents, but it is believed that females are under-diagnosed. Approximately 8–10 % of males, and 3–4 % of females, under the age of 18 have ADHD. Roughly 80 % of children with ADHD will continue to meet diagnostic criteria for ADHD into their adolescent years and 60 % will maintain core symptoms into adulthood (Wittchen et al. 2011; Dopheide and Pliszka 2009; Weyandt and Dupaul 2008).

In the international scientific literature, prevalence estimates vary widely across studies. At one extreme, in Colombia, the prevalence rates were estimated to be 19 and 12 % for boys and girls respectively; combined type 6.4 %, inattentive type 4.8 %, and hyperactive impulsive type 3 % (Pineda et al. 2003). Such a wide range in prevalence estimates is unlikely to reflect true differences in the numbers of individuals with ADHD in various populations. Polanczyk and colleagues (2008) conducted a systematic review of prevalence studies and concluded that the great majority of variability stemmed from the methods used, such as the way symptoms were measured and the exact definitions used. There were relatively minor differences in different parts of the world and the review's summary of rates was around 5.3 % (Polanczyk and Jensen 2008).

3.2 Etiology

The etiology of ADHD involves the interplay of multiple genetic and environmental factors. There is no one direct cause for ADHD, either genetic or non-genetic. Rather, it is the complex interactions of multiple genes and multiple environmental risk factors.

J. Sadek, *A Clinician's Guide to ADHD*,
DOI 10.1007/978-3-319-02359-5_3,

- **Genetic**
  There is robust evidence from studies of a strong inherited contribution to ADHD. This finding is supported by twin studies, adoption studies, family studies and molecular genetics studies. There is no one direct cause for ADHD, either genetic or non-genetic. Rather, it is the complex interactions of multiple genes and multiple environmental risk factors that contribute to the development of this disorder. ADHD is highly heritable disorder but the rate is not 100 %. It has been reported in some studies as high as 79 %. ADHD shares an inherited liability with developmental coordination problems, reading ability, IQ, mood and conduct problems (Sharp et al. 2009; Martin et al. 2008; Sprich et al 2000; Paloyelis et al. 2010; Cole et al. 2009; Thapar et al. 2001).
- **Susceptibility Genes**
  Abnormalities in the dopamine D4 and D5 receptor genes (DRD 4 & DRD5) are associated with ADHD. Dopamine transporter genes (DAT1) lead to low levels of dopamine in the brain in patients with ADHD (Faraone et al. 2001, 2005; Li et al. 2006; DiMaio et al. 2003).
  Some rare genetic disorders, deletion syndromes and chromosomal anomalies are associated with ADHD. Examples include neurofibromatosis type 1, Angelman, Prader-Willi, Fragile X syndrome, Tuberous Sclerosis and 22 q 11 microdeletion (Elia et al. 2009; Lesch et al 2011; Williams et al. 2010).
- **Neuroimaging and Neurochemistry**
  ADHD is thought to result from hypoactive frontal cortex and subcortical structures that decrease the production of dopamine and norepinephrine. Neuroimaging studies confirm that brain abnormalities in frontosubcortical networks are associated with ADHD but neuroimaging techniques are not valid tools for ADHD diagnosis; imaging measures are not sensitive or specific enough to be used for diagnostic purposes.
  Dorsal ACC (Anterior Cingulate Cortex) has been associated with selective attention (details, listen, loose, forget). Prefrontal PF motor cortex has been associated with hyperactivity symptoms. Orbitofrontal Cortex has been associated with impulsive symptoms. Dorsolateral Prefrontal Cortex (DLPFC) has been linked to problem solving, sustained attention and executive function (organization, follow through, avoiding sustained mental effort).
  Neuroimaging and MRI studies of children with ADHD have reported abnormalities in the prefrontal cortex and basal ganglia, reduced size of the frontal cortex, cerebellum, basal ganglia, corpus Callosum and frontal lobes. Hypoperfusion was also reported in the striatum (Connor et al. 2010; Rösler et al. 2010; Thapar et al. 2012; Frodl and Skokauskas 2012; Castellanos and Proal 2012; Liston et al. 2011; Bush 2011).
- **Pregnancy and early childhood factors**
  Several factors have shown clinical and epidemiological association with ADHD. These include maternal cigarette smoking and alcohol consumption that lead to fetal alcohol syndrome or street drug use (such as heroin) during pregnancy. It was also suggested that very low birth weight, prematurity, fetal hypoxia and brain injury may predispose to ADHD. Maternal stress during pregnancy has

also been associated with ADHD (Keenan et al. 2008; Langley et al. 2005; Mick et al. 2002; Rice et al. 2010; Aarnoudse-Moens et al. 2009).

- **Toxins and Dietary factors**

  Exposure to toxins such as pesticides, polychlorinated biphenyl (PCBs), led and deficiency of iron and zinc were studied in attempt to understand their contributions to ADHD.

  Food additives, sugar, coloring agent, omega 3 fatty acids and elimination die have been studied in relation to ADHD symptoms. Recent randomized clinical trial showed some benefit in using elimination diet in improving ADHD symptoms. More studies are being conducted on the benefit of omega-3 long chain polyunsaturated fatty acids (PUFA) in improving symptoms of ADHD (Nigg 2008; Bouchard et al. 2010; Eubig et al. 2010; Ballard et al. 2010; Pelsser et al. 2011).
- **Psychosocial factors**

  ADHD has been associated with severe early psychosocial adversity. Low parental education, poverty, deprivation, negative parenting, bullying, peer victimization, family discord are associated with ADHD (Lifford et al. 2008; Kreppner et al. 2010; Ficks and Waldman 2009).

References

Aarnoudse-Moens CSH, Weisglas-Kuperus N, van Goudoever JB, Oosterlaan J (2009) Meta-analysis of neurobehavioral outcomes in very preterm and/or very low birth weight children. Pediatrics 124(2):717–728

Ballard W, Hall MN, Kaufmann L (2010) Do dietary interventions improve ADHD symptoms in children? Clin Inq 59:234–235 (MU)

Bouchard MF, Bellinger DC, Wright RO, Weisskopf MG (2010) Attention-deficit/hyperactivity disorder and urinary metabolites of organophosphate pesticides. Pediatrics 125(6):e1270–e1277

Bush G (2011) Cingulate, frontal, and parietal cortical dysfunction in attention-deficit/hyperactivity disorder. Biol Psychiatry 69(12):1160–1167

Castellanos FX, Proal E (2012) Large-scale brain systems in ADHD: beyond the prefrontal–striatal model. Trends Cogn Sci 16(1):17–26

Cole J, Ball HA, Martin NC, Scourfield J, Mcguffin P (2009) Genetic overlap between measures of hyperactivity/inattention and mood in children and adolescents. J Am Acad Child Adolesc Psychiatry 48(11):1094–1101

Connor DF, Steeber J, McBurnett K (2010) A review of attention-deficit/hyperactivity disorder complicated by symptoms of oppositional defiant disorder or conduct disorder. J Dev Behav Pediatr 31(5):427–440

DiMaio S, Grizenko N, Joober R (2003) Dopamine genes and attention-deficit hyperactivity disorder: a review. J Psychiatry Neurosci 28(1):27–38

Dopheide JA, Pliszka SR (2009) Attention deficit hyperactivity disorder: an update. Pharmacotherapy 29(6):656–679

Elia J, Gai X, Xie HM, Perin JC, Geiger E, Glessner JT, D'arcy M (2009) Rare structural variants found in attention-deficit hyperactivity disorder are preferentially associated with neurodevelopmental genes. Mol Psychiatry 15(6):637–646

Eubig PA, Aguiar A, Schantz SL (2010) Lead and PCBs as risk factors for attention deficit/hyperactivity disorder. Environ Health Perspect 118(12):1654

Faraone SV, Doyle AE, Mick E, Biederman J (2001) Meta-analysis of the association between the 7-repeat allele of the dopamine D4 receptor gene and attention deficit hyperactivity disorder. Am J Psychiatry 158(7):1052–1057

Faraone SV, Perlis RH, Doyle AE, Smoller JW, Goralnick JJ, Holmgren MA, Sklar P (2005) Molecular genetics of attention-deficit/hyperactivity disorder. Biol Psychiatry 57(11): 1313–1323
Ficks CA, Waldman ID (2009) Gene-environment interactions in attention-deficit/hyperactivity disorder. Curr Psychiatry Rep 11(5):387–392
Frodl T, Skokauskas N (2012) Meta analysis of structural MRI studies in children and adults with attention deficit hyperactivity disorder indicates treatment effects. Acta Psychiatr Scand 125(2):114–126
Keenan HT, Hall GC, Marshall SW (2008) Early head injury and attention deficit hyperactivity disorder: retrospective cohort study. BMJ 337:a1984
Kreppner J, Kumsta R, Rutter M, Beckett C, Castle J, Stevens S, Sonuga Barke EJ (2010) IV. Developmental course of deprivation specific psychological patterns: early manifestations, persistence to age 15, and clinical features. Monogr Soc Res Child Dev 75(1):79–101
Langley K, Rice F, Van den Bree MB, Thapar A (2005) Maternal smoking during pregnancy as an environmental risk factor for attention deficit hyperactivity disorder behaviour. A review. Minerva Pediatr 57(6):359–371
Lesch KP, Selch S, Renner TJ, Jacob C, Nguyen TT, Hahn T et al (2011) Genome-wide copy number variation analysis in attention-deficit/hyperactivity disorder: association with neuropeptide Y gene dosage in an extended pedigree. Mol Psychiatry 16(5):491–503
Li D, Sham PC, Owen MJ, He L (2006) Meta-analysis shows significant association between dopamine system genes and attention deficit hyperactivity disorder (ADHD). Hum Mol Genet 15(14):2276–2284
Lifford KJ, Harold GT, Thapar A (2008) Parent–child relationships and ADHD symptoms: a longitudinal analysis. J Abnorm Child Psychol 36(2):285–296
Liston C, Cohen MM, Teslovich T, Levenson D, Casey BJ (2011) Atypical prefrontal connectivity in attention-deficit/hyperactivity disorder: pathway to disease or pathological end point? Biol Psychiatry 69(12):1168–1177
Martin N, McDougall M, Hay DA (2008) What are the key directions in the genetics of attention deficit hyperactivity disorder? Curr Opin Psychiatry 21(4):356–361
Mick E, Biederman J, Faraone SV, Sayer J, Kleinman S (2002) Case-control study of attention-deficit hyperactivity disorder and maternal smoking, alcohol use, and drug use during pregnancy. J Am Acad Child Adolesc Psychiatry 41(4):378–385
Nigg JT (2008) ADHD, lead exposure and prevention: how much lead or how much evidence is needed? Expert Rev Neurother 8(4):519–521
Paloyelis Y, Rijsdijk F, Wood AC, Asherson P, Kuntsi J (2010) The genetic association between ADHD symptoms and reading difficulties: the role of inattentiveness and IQ. J Abnorm Child Psychol 38(8):1083–1095
Pelsser LM, Frankena K, Toorman J, Savelkoul HF, Dubois AE, Pereira RR et al (2011) Effects of a restricted elimination diet on the behaviour of children with attention-deficit hyperactivity disorder (INCA study): a randomised controlled trial. Lancet 377(9764):494–503
Pineda DA, Lopera F, Palacio JD, Ramirez D, Henao GC (2003) Prevalence estimations of attention-deficit/hyperactivity disorder: differential diagnoses and comorbidities in a Colombian sample. Int J Neurosci 113(1):49–71
Polanczyk G, Jensen P (2008) Epidemiologic considerations in attention deficit hyperactivity disorder: a review and update. Child Adolesc Psychiatr Clin N Am 17(2):245–260
Rice F, Harold GT, Boivin J, Van den Bree M, Hay DF, Thapar A (2010) The links between prenatal stress and offspring development and psychopathology: disentangling environmental and inherited influences. Psychol Med 40(02):335–345
Rösler M, Retz W, Stieglitz RD (2010) Psychopathological rating scales as efficacy parameters in adult ADHD treatment investigations-benchmarking instruments for international multicentre trials. Pharmacopsychiatry 43(03):92–98
Sharp SI, McQuillin A, Gurling H (2009) Genetics of attention-deficit hyperactivity disorder (ADHD). Neuropharmacology 57(7):590–600

Sprich S, Biederman J, Crawford MH, Mundy E, Faraone SV (2000) Adoptive and biological families of children and adolescents with ADHD. J Am Acad Child Adolesc Psychiatry 39(11):1432–1437

Thapar A, Harrington R, McGuffin P (2001) Examining the comorbidity of ADHD-related behaviours and conduct problems using a twin study design. Br J Psychiatry 179(3):224–229

Thapar A, Cooper M, Jefferies R, Stergiakouli E (2012) What causes attention deficit hyperactivity disorder? Arch Dis Child 97(3):260–265

Weyandt LL, DuPaul GJ (2008) ADHD in college students: developmental findings. Dev Disabil Res Rev 14(4):311–319

Williams NM, Zaharieva I, Martin A, Langley K, Mantripragada K, Fossdal R et al (2010) Rare chromosomal deletions and duplications in attention-deficit hyperactivity disorder: a genome-wide analysis. Lancet 376(9750):1401–1408

Wittchen HU, Jacobi F, Rehm J, Gustavsson A, Svensson M, Jönsson B et al (2011) The size and burden of mental disorders and other disorders of the brain in Europe 2010. Eur Neuropsychopharmacol 21(9):655–679

ADHD Guidelines Available on the Internet

American Psychological Association. http://www.apa.org/topics/adhd/index.aspx

Australian ADHD Draft Guidelines. http://www.nhmrc.gov.au/guidelines/publications/ch54

Canadian ADHD Guidelines. http://www.caddra.ca/cms4/

National Institute for Health and Clinical Excellence (NICE). http://publications.nice.org.uk/attention-deficit-hyperactivity-disorder-cg72

Scottish ADHD Guidelines. http://www.sign.ac.uk/guidelines/fulltext/112/index.html

Impairment in Patients with ADHD

4

Please refer to the back of the book where scales are provided for the Weiss scale which identifies impairments.

4.1 Impairment in Children with ADHD

Children with ADHD typically underachieve academically, repeat grades, drop out of school, have difficulties with peer relationships, disrupt family functioning, and are more likely than their peers without ADHD to be delinquent and be more accident prone (Barkley 2006).

In adolescents, higher rates of school suspensions and dropouts, conduct disorder and oppositional defiant disorder, teenage pregnancy, sexually transmitted diseases, and increased rates of substance use have been found (Brown and Pacini 1989; Barkley et al. 2006).

4.2 Impairment in Adults with ADHD

Here some of the important areas of functioning that may be impaired by ADHD: occupational, academic, and family/social/emotional/interpersonal functioning impairments. Please refer to the chapter *ADHD and Driving* specifically referring to the unique issues of driving impairment for individuals with ADHD.

- **Occupational functioning**
  There is a growing body of evidence that argues that symptoms of deficient executive functioning (EF) may also be involved in attention deficit hyperactivity disorder (ADHD) (Barkley 1997, 2001; Castellanos et al. 2006).
  Adult occupational functioning would be expected to be influenced by EF. This can be explained by the need for organization and maintenance of behavior and problem-solving toward goals across days, weeks, or even months. Effective performance at work requires the capacity for self-management relative to time (time management), self-organization planning and problem-solving,

J. Sadek, *A Clinician's Guide to ADHD*,

DOI 10.1007/978-3-319-02359-5_4,

self-activation, and self-motivation to sustain the pursuit of larger delayed consequences over smaller more immediate ones (deferred gratification), among other activities, that are presumed to be facilitated by the EFs (Barkley and Murphy 2010).

Increasing evidence indicates that adult ADHD is associated with the following problems:

Barkley et al. in 2008 note:

- individuals rank significantly lower than control groups in occupational status;
- individuals may have significantly worse job performance ratings from employers;
- adults with ADHD may be more likely fired from employment and to be so more often.

Mentioned each by DeQuiros and Kinsbourne 2001; Halmoy et al. 2009; Murphy and Barkley 1996 are these impairments:

adults are more likely to be unemployed;

individuals are more likely to be fired from employment or impulsively quit a job;

individuals may use more sick time, which might further lead to applying for and needing disability pension;

adults may change jobs impulsively more often.

Painter, Prevatte and Welles in 2008 note:

- adults with ADHD also appear to have more dysfunctional career beliefs;
- decision making can be confusing for them;
- individuals experience greater work-related anxiety and external conflict regarding their careers.

Finally, de Graaf et al. in 2008 note:

- significantly more "days out" of role or under productive;
- there is more than twice the risk of absence due to sickness, and;
- more than twice the risk of workplace accidents that other working adults.

- **Academic impairment**

  Adults with ADHD function fall below their ability for most of their lives. They are faced with several academic difficulties. Some examples are:

  - Despite high IQs in some patients with ADHD, they may experience difficulty completing college or achieving career milestones (Nadeau 2005).
  - Grade retention and a higher rate of suspension or expulsion from school exists (Adler and Cohen 2004).
  - Less likelihood of graduating from high school or obtaining a college degree (Biederman et al. 2006).
  - A three-fold increased likelihood of failing a grade or suspension and an eight-fold increased likelihood of school expulsion or dropout among adolescents who were diagnosed with ADHD in childhood as compared with adolescents without ADHD (Barkley et al. 1990).

- **Family, social, emotional and interpersonal functioning**
  The chronic disabling nature of ADHD significantly increased the likelihood of psychiatric, social, legal and family problems in adulthood. ADHD can reduce the quality of life significantly. The following problems were reported in the literature:
  - Poor social functioning and difficulty relating to others (Clarke et al. 2005)
  - Tension in the family (Adler and Cohen 2004)
  - Poor day-to-day supervision of their children including treatment regimens – and confound many family activities (Adler and Cohen 2004)
  - Poor relationships with parents and children and poor parenting skills (Biederman et al. 2006)
  - Strained or unstable relationships with significant others and poor perceptions of their ability to provide emotional support (5)
  - Poor ability of the adult with ADHD to sort out problems when they arise (Adler and Cohen 2004)
  - Not fitting in with peers, not liked by other adults, and a greater tendency toward anti-social behavior (Biederman et al. 2006)
  - Poor self-esteem (Adler and Cohen 2004)
  - Chaotic personal and family life (divorces, moves) (Adler and Cohen 2004)
  - Increased risk of adult criminal activity and incarceration (Babinski et al. 1999)
  - More arrests and self-reported crimes (Babinski et al. 1999)
  - Participation in more serious crimes (Eyestone and Howell 1994)
  - Substance abuse and dependence (Wilens 2004)
  - More economic burden to patient and family (Swensen et al. 2004)
  - Poor financial management (Secnik et al. 2005)
  - More sexually transmitted disease, more promiscuous behavior and more teen pregnancy (Fowler et al. 2009)

References

Adler L, Cohen J (2004) Diagnosis and evaluation of adults with attention-deficit/hyperactivity disorder. Psychiatr Clin N Am 27(2):187–201

Babinski LM, Hartsough CS, Lambert NM (1999) Childhood conduct problems, hyperactivity impulsivity, and inattention as predictors of adult criminal activity. J Child Psychol Psychiatry 40(3):347–355

Barkley RA (2006) Attention deficit hyperactivity disorder: handbook for diagnosis and treatment, 3rd edn. The Guildford Press, New York

Barkley RA (2001) The inattentive type of ADHD as a distinct disorder: what remains to be done. Clin Psychol Sci Pract 8(4):489–493

Barkley RA (1997) Behavioral inhibition, sustained attention, and executive functions: constructing a unifying theory of ADHD. Psychol Bull 121(1):65–94

Barkley RA, Murphy KR (2010) Impairment in occupational functioning and adult ADHD: the predictive utility of executive function (EF) ratings versus EF tests. Arch Clin Neuropsychol 25(3):157–173

Barkley RA, Murphy KR, Fischer M (2008) ADHD in adults: what the science says. Guilford Press, New York

Barkley RA, Fischer M, Smallish L, Fletcher K (2006) Young adult outcome of hyperactive children: adaptive functioning in major life activities. J Am Acad Child Adolesc Psychiatry 45(2):192–202
Barkley RA, Fischer M, Edelbrock CS, Smallish L (1990) The adolescent outcome of hyperactive children diagnosed by research criteria: I. An 8-year prospective follow-up study. J Am Acad Child Adolesc Psychiatry 29(4):546–557
Biederman J, Faraone SV, Spencer TJ, Mick E, Monuteaux MC, Aleardi M (2006) Functional impairments in adults with self-reports of diagnosed ADHD: a controlled study of 1001 adults in the community. J Clin Psychiatry 67:524–540
Brown RT, Pacini JN (1989) Perceived family functioning, marital status, and depression in parents of boys with attention deficit disorder. J Learn Disabil 22(9):581–587
Castellanos FX, Sonuga-Barke EJ, Milham MP, Tannock R (2006) Characterizing cognition in ADHD: beyond executive dysfunction. Trends Cogn Sci 10(3):117–123
Clarke S, Heussler H, Kohn MR (2005) Attention deficit disorder: not just for children. Intern Med J 35(12):721–725
De Graaf R, Kessler RC, Fayyad J, ten Have M, Alonso J, Angermeyer M et al (2008) The prevalence and effects of adult attention-deficit/hyperactivity disorder (ADHD) on the performance of workers: results from the WHO World Mental Health Survey Initiative. Occup Environ Med 65(12):835–842
DeQuiros GB, Kinsbourne M (2001) Adult ADHD: analysis of self-ratings on a behavior questionnaire. In: Wasserstein J, Wolf L, Lefever F (eds) Adult attention deficit disorder: brain mechanisms and life outcomes, vol 931, Annals of the New York Academy of sciences. New York Academy of Sciences, New York, pp 140–147
Fowler T, Langley K, Rice F, Whittinger N, Ross K, van Goozen S et al (2009) Psychopathy traits in adolescents with childhood attention-deficit hyperactivity disorder. Br J Psychiatry 194(1):62–67
Eyestone LL, Howell RJ (1994) An epidemiological study of attention-deficit hyperactivity disorder and major depression in a male prison population. J Am Acad Psychiatry Law Online 22(2):181–193
Halmoy A, Fasmer OB, Gillberg C, Haavik J (2009) Occupational outcome in adult ADHD: impact of symptom profile, comorbid psychiatric problems, and treatment a cross-sectional study of 414 clinically diagnosed adult ADHD patients. J Atten Disord 13(2):175–187
Murphy K, Barkley RA (1996) Attention deficit hyperactivity disorder adults: comorbidities and adaptive impairments. Compr Psychiatry 37(6):393–401
Nadeau KG (2005) Career choices and workplace challenges for individuals with ADHD. J Clin Psychol 61(5):549–563
Painter CA, Prevatt F, Welles T (2008) Career beliefs and job satisfaction in adults with symptoms of attention deficit/hyperactivity disorder. J Employ Couns 45(4):178–188
Secnik K, Swensen A, Lage MJ (2005) Comorbidities and costs of adult patients diagnosed with attention-deficit hyperactivity disorder. Pharmacoeconomics 23(1):93–102
Swensen A, Birnbaum HG, Ben Hamadi R, Greenberg P, Cremieux PY, Secnik K (2004) Incidence and costs of accidents among attention-deficit/hyperactivity disorder patients. J Adolesc Health 35(4):346-e1
Wilens TE (2004) Attention-deficit/hyperactivity disorder and the substance use disorders: the nature of the relationship, subtypes at risk, and treatment issues. Psychiatr Clin N Am 27(2):283–301

Other References and Recommended Readings

Alderman N, Burgess PW, Knight C, Henman C (2003) Ecological validity a simplified version of the multiple errands shopping test. J Int Neuropsychol Soc 9:31–44

Barkley RA (2006) Attention deficit hyperactivity disorder: handbook for diagnosis and treatment, 3rd edn. The Guildford Press, New York (also workbook)

Barkley RA, Fischer M (2010) Predicting impairment in major life activities and occupational functioning in hyperactive children as adults: self-reported executive function (EF) deficits vs. EF tests. Dev Neuropsychol 36(2):137–161

Barkley RA, Murphy KR (2010) Impairment in occupational functioning and adult ADHD: the predictive utility of executive function (EF) ratings versus EF tests. Arch Clin Neuropsychol 5(3):157–173

Barkley RA, Fischer M, Smallish L et al (2004) Young adult follow-up of hyperactive children: antisocial activities and drug use. J Child Psychol Psychiatry 45:195–211

Barkley RA, Fischer M, Smallish L et al (2006) Young adult outcome of hyperactive children: adaptive functioning in major life activities. J Am Acad Child Adolesc Psychiatry 45(2):192–202

Barkley RA, Murphy KR, Fischer M (2008b) ADHD in adults: what the science says. Guilford, New York

Biederman J, Faraone S (2005) Attention-deficit hyperactivity disorder. Lancet 366:237–248

Biederman J, Faraone SV (2006) The effects of attention-deficit/hyperactivity disorder on employment and household income. MedGenMed 8:12

Biederman J, Petty CR, Fried R, Black S, Faneuil A, Doyle AE et al (2008) Discordance between psychometric testing and questionnaire-based definitions of executive function deficits in individuals with ADHD. J Atten Disord 12:92–102

Brown TE (1996) Brown attention-deficit disorder scales. The Psychological Corporation, San Antonio

Faraone S, Biederman J, Mick E (2005) The age-dependent decline of attention deficit hyperactivity disorder: a meta-analysis of follow-up studies. Psychol Med 35:1–7

Frazier TW, Demareem HA, Youngstrom EA (2004) Meta-analysis of intellectual and neuropsychological test performance in attention-deficit/hyperactivity disorder. Neuropsychology 18:543–555

Kessler RC, Adler L, Barkley RA, Biederman J, Conners CK, Demler O et al (2006) The prevalence and correlates of adult ADHD in the United States: results from the National Comorbidity Survey Replication. Am J Psychiatry 163:716–723

Mannuzza S, Klein RG, Bessler A et al (1997) Educational and occupational outcome of hyperactive boys grown up. J Am Acad Child Adolesc Psychiatry 36:1222–1227

Mao AR. A physician's guide to helping patients with ADHD Find success in the workplace. Postgrad Med

Mao AR, Brams M, Babcock T, Madhoo M (2011) A physician's guide to helping patients with ADHD find success in the workplace. Postgrad Med 123(5):60–70

Matza LS, Paramore C, Prasad M (2005) A review of the economic burden of ADHD. Cost Eff Resour Alloc 3:5

McGough JJ, Barkley RA (2004) Diagnostic controversies in adult attention deficit hyperactivity disorder. Am J Psychiatry 161:1948–1956

Nigg JT, Wilcutt EG, Doyle AE, Sonuga-Barke JS (2005) Causal heterogeneity in attention-deficit/hyperactivity disorder: do we need neuropsychologically impaired subtypes? Biol Psychiatry 57:1224–1230

Palacio JD, Castellanos FX, Pineda DA et al (2004) Attention-deficit/hyperactivity disorder and comorbidities in 18 Paisa Colombian multigenerational families. J Am Acad Child Adolesc Psychiatry 43:1506–1515

Riccio C, Wolfe M, Davis B et al (2005) Attention deficit hyperactivity disorder: manifestation in adulthood. Arch Clin Neuropsychol 20:249–269

Weiss M, Weiss J (2004) A guide to the treatment of adults with ADHD. J Clin Psychiatry 65(3):27–37

Wilens T, Dodson W (2004) A clinical perspective of attention-deficit/hyperactivity disorder into adulthood. J Clin Psychiatry 65:1301–1313

Wilens T, Gignac M, Swezey A et al (2006) Characteristics of adolescents and young adults with ADHD who divert or misuse their prescribed medications. J Am Acad Child Adolesc Psychiatry 45:408–414

Young S, Toone B, Tyson C (2003) Comorbidity and psychosocial profile of adults with attention deficit hyperactivity disorder. Pers Individ Differ 35:743–755

ADHD Guidelines Available on the Internet

American Psychological Association. http://www.apa.org/topics/adhd/index.aspx

Australian ADHD Draft Guidelines. http://www.nhmrc.gov.au/guidelines/publications/ch54

Canadian ADHD Guidelines. http://www.caddra.ca/cms4/

National Institute for Health and Clinical Excellence (NICE). http://publications.nice.org.uk/attention-deficit-hyperactivity-disorder-cg72

Scottish ADHD Guidelines. http://www.sign.ac.uk/guidelines/fulltext/112/index.html

How to Diagnose ADHD in Children and Adolescents

5

1. Identify your patients: 3–18 year old patient identified with signs or symptoms suggesting ADHD. Symptoms can come from parents' direct concerns, or the mental health screen, or school, or other sources in group homes or institutions.
2. Review with the parents and patient their concerns, reason for referral, and the parents' and patient's (in the case of older children or adolescents) hopes for the assessment. Clarify if the symptoms have been present since the patient was young, and at what age they think the symptoms started, and how it progressed. Ask the parents, or patient, to bring all past documentation (e.g., school report cards, assessments, etc.). Obtain written consent to release information for institutional documentation. It is suggested that asking for documentation can be done by phone prior to the interview.
3. Obtain past psychiatric history and any prior ADHD diagnosis, medical history, family history of ADHD and other psychiatric and medical disorders.
4. Obtain the psychosocial history including pregnancy, birth history, developmental milestones, school performance, learning problems, parenting, abuse (both sexual and physical), temperament, relationship with others at home and at school, defiance and oppositional behavior, conduct related problems, and ask about current stressors and current medications.
5. Review of systems would include basic screening for comorbidities or presence of other disorders as mood disorder, anxiety disorder, learning disorders, sleeping problems, tics, seizure disorders, and substance abuse in adolescents.
6. Document that a physical examination was completed with an emphasis on hearing, vision, weight and neurological exam. Review routine blood work, including TSH. Ensure that there are no other medical causes of the symptoms of ADHD. Ensure that there are no medical contraindications to the use of medications for the treatment of ADHD symptoms.

J. Sadek, *A Clinician's Guide to ADHD*,
DOI 10.1007/978-3-319-02359-5_5,

7. Use rating scales and questionnaires (some are available at www.caddra.ca). Refer to the list of scales in the Reference section of this book to select what scales you want to use. They are an efficient way to obtain information from the patient and get collateral sources mainly from parents and teachers. They should be updated over time. Clinical judgment is mandatory for the interpretation of the results of these scales and questionnaires. Use the DSM-IV criteria to verify if the patient fulfills DSM- IV criteria, or not.

5.1 Diagnostic Criteria According to DSM-IV – Children

Text below (in italics) is a direct reproduction of text from DSM-IV TR. Please refer to the copyright page at the beginning of the book for further reference.

A. ***Symptoms either (1) or (2)***

(1) Six (or more) of the following symptoms of ***inattention*** *nave persisted for at least 6 months to a degree that is maladaptive and inconsistent with developmental levels.*	*(2) Six (or more) of the following symptoms of* hyperactivity-impulsivity *have persisted for at least 6 months to a degree that is maladaptive and inconsistent with developmental levels.*
Inattention	***Hyperactivity***
a) often fails to give close attention to details or makes careless mistakes in schoolwork, work or other activities	*a) often fidgets with hands or feet or squirms in seat*
b) often has difficulty sustaining attention in tasks or play activities	*b) often leaves seat in classroom or in other situations in which remaining seated is expected*
c) often does not seem to listen when spoken to directly	*c) often runs about or climbs excessively in situations in which it is inappropriate (in adolescents or adults, may be limited to subjective feelings of restlessness*
d) often does not follow through on instructions and fails to finish schoolwork, chores, or duties in the workplace (not due to oppositional behavior or failure to understand instructions)	*d) often has difficulty playing or engaging in leisure activities quietly*
e) often has difficulty organizing tasks and activities	*e) often is "on the go" or often acts as if "driven by a motor"*
f) often avoids, dislikes, or is reluctant to engage in tasks that require sustained mental effort (such as schoolwork of homework)	*f) often talks excessively.*
g) often loses things necessary for tasks or activities (e.g. toys, school assignments, pencils, books or tools)	***Impulsivity***
h) often is easily distracted by extraneous stimuli	*g) often blurts out answers before questions have been completed;*
i) often is forgetful in daily activities	*h) often has difficulty awaiting turn;* *i) often interrupts or intrudes on others (e.g. butts into conversations or games)*

B. *Some hyperactive-impulsive or inattentive symptoms that cause impairment were present before age 7 years (DSM V is age 12).*
C. *Some impairment from the symptoms is present in two or more settings (e.g. at school [or work], and at home).*
D. *There must be clear evidence of clinically significant impairment in social, academic, or occupational functioning.*
E. *The symptoms do not occur exclusively during the course of a Schizophrenia, or other Psychotic Disorder, and are not better accounted for by another mental disorder (e.g. Mood Disorder, Anxiety Disorder, Dissociative Disorder, or a Personality Disorder).*

Code base on type

314.01 Attention-Deficit/Hyperactivity Disorder, combined type: if both Criteria A1 –A2 are met for the past 6 months.

314.00 Attention-Deficit/Hyperactivity Disorder, Predominantly Inattentive type: if Criterion A1 is met but Criterion A2 is not for the past 6 months.

314.00 Attention-Deficit/Hyperactivity Disorder, Predominantly Hyperactivity-Impulsive type: if Criterion A2 is met but Criterion A1 is not for the past 6 months.

ADHD Guidelines Available on the Internet

American Psychological Association. http://www.apa.org/topics/adhd/index.aspx
Australian ADHD Draft Guidelines. http://www.nhmrc.gov.au/guidelines/publications/ch54
Canadian ADHD Guidelines. http://www.caddra.ca/cms4/
National Institute for Health and Clinical Excellence (NICE). http://publications.nice.org.uk/attention-deficit-hyperactivity-disorder-cg72
Scottish ADHD Guidelines. http://www.sign.ac.uk/guidelines/fulltext/112/index.html

How to Diagnose ADHD in Adults

6

1. Review with the patient (and the significant other or family member if possible) their concerns, reason for referral, and the patient's hopes for the assessment. Clarify if the symptoms have been present since the patient was young, and at what age they think the symptoms started, and how it progressed. Ask the patient to bring all past documentation (e.g. school report cards, assessments, etc.). Obtain written consent to release information for institutional documentation. It is suggested that asking for documentation can be done by phone prior to the interview.
2. Obtain past psychiatric history and any prior ADHD diagnosis, medical history, family history of ADHD and other psychiatric and medical disorders.
3. Obtain the psychosocial history including complications during mother's pregnancy with patient, birth history, developmental milestones, school performance, learning problems, parenting, abuse both sexual and physical, temperament, relationship with others at home and in the past at school, defiance and oppositional behavior, conduct related problems, and ask about current stressors and current medications. Ask about work history and problems at work. As about marital and relationship difficulties and obtain sexual history. Ask about problems with the law.
4. Review of systems would include basic screening for comorbidities or presence of other disorders as mood disorder, anxiety disorder, somatoform disorder, learning disorders, sleeping problems, tics, seizure disorders, and personality disorder.
5. Document that a physical examination was completed with an emphasis on neurological exam. Review routine blood work, including TSH. Ensure that there are no other medical causes of the symptoms of ADHD. Ensure that there are no medical contraindications to the use of medications for the treatment of ADHD symptoms.
6. Use rating scales and questionnaires (some are available at www.caddra.ca). Scales are efficient way to obtain information from the patient and collateral sources mainly partner and family. They should be updated over time. Clinical judgment is mandatory for the interpretation of the results of these scales and questionnaires. Use the DSM-V criteria to verify if the patient fulfills ADHD criteria, or not.

J. Sadek, *A Clinician's Guide to ADHD*,
DOI 10.1007/978-3-319-02359-5_6,

6.1 Diagnostic Criteria in Adults

Text below (in italics) is a direct reproduction of text from DSM-IV TR and some of the changes in DSM-V. Please refer to the copyright page at the beginning of the book for further reference.

A. ***Symptoms either (1) or (2)***

(1) Five (or more) of the following symptoms of ***inattention*** *have persisted for at least 6 months to a degree that is maladaptive and inconsistent with developmental levels (used to be six in DSM-IV).*	*(2) Five (or more) of the following symptoms of* hyperactivity-impulsivity *have persisted for at least 6 months to a degree that is maladaptive and inconsistent with developmental levels (used to be six in DSM-IV).*
Inattention	***Hyperactivity***
a) often fails to give close attention to details or makes careless mistakes in schoolwork, work or other activities	*a) often fidgets with hands or feet or squirms in seat*
b) often has difficulty sustaining attention in tasks or play activities	*b) often leaves seat in classroom or in other situations in which remaining seated is expected*
c) often does not seem to listen when spoken to directly	*c) often runs about or climbs excessively in situations in which it is inappropriate (in adolescents or adults, may be limited to subjective feelings of restlessness*
d) often does not follow through on instructions and fails to finish schoolwork, chores, or duties in the workplace (not due to oppositional behavior or failure to understand instructions)	*d) often has difficulty playing or engaging in leisure activities quietly*
e) often has difficulty organizing tasks and activities	*e) often is "on the go" or often acts as if "driven by a motor"*
f) often avoids, dislikes, or is reluctant to engage in tasks that require sustained mental effort (such as schoolwork or homework)	*f) often talks excessively.*
g) often loses things necessary for tasks or activities (e.g. toys, school assignments, pencils, books or tools)	***Impulsivity***
h) often is easily distracted by extraneous stimuli	*g) often blurts out answers before questions have been completed;*
i) is forgetful in daily activities.	*h) often has difficulty awaiting turn;* *i) often interrupts or intrudes on others (e.g. butts into conversations or games).*

B. *Some hyperactive-impulsive or inattentive symptoms that cause impairment were present before age 7 years (age 12 now).*

C. *Some impairment from the symptoms is present in two or more settings (e.g. at school [or work], and at home).*

D. *There must be clear evidence of clinically significant impairment in social, academic, or occupational functioning.*

E. *The symptoms do not occur exclusively during the course of Psychotic Disorders, and are not better accounted for by another mental disorder (e.g. Mood Disorder, Anxiety Disorder, Dissociative Disorder, or a Personality Disorder).*

Code base on type

314.01 Attention-Deficit/Hyperactivity Disorder, combined type: if both Criteria A1 –A2 are met for the past 6 months.

314.00 Attention-Deficit/Hyperactivity Disorder, Predominantly Inattentive type: if Criterion A1 is met but Criterion A2 is not for the past 6 months.

314.00 Attention-Deficit/Hyperactivity Disorder, Predominantly Hyperactivity-Impulsive type: if Criterion A2 is met but Criterion A1 is not for the past 6 months.

6.2 Other Common Impulsivity Symptoms for Adults

- often acts without thinking (e.g. starting jobs without adequate preparation, making decisions without thinking, sudden job changes)
- is often impatient (e.g. traffic violations and cutting through traffic)
- often ignores to do activities carefully or properly so the results are rushed and defective at times)
- often has difficulty pressure, temptations or opportunities that should not be accepted.

ADHD Guidelines Available on the Internet

American Psychological Association. http://www.apa.org/topics/adhd/index.aspx
Australian ADHD Draft Guidelines. http://www.nhmrc.gov.au/guidelines/publications/ch54
Canadian ADHD Guidelines. http://www.caddra.ca/cms4/
National Institute for Health and Clinical Excellence (NICE). http://publications.nice.org.uk/attention-deficit-hyperactivity-disorder-cg72
Scottish ADHD Guidelines. http://www.sign.ac.uk/guidelines/fulltext/112/index.html

7 Differential Diagnosis

1. **Differential Diagnosis**: **Psychiatric Conditions AXIS I**:
    1.1. Bipolar Disorder
    1.2. Learning or language disorder
    1.3. Major Depression
    1.4. Anxiety Disorder
    1.5. Conduct Disorder/Oppositional Defiant Disorder
    1.6. Obsessive Compulsive Disorder
    1.7. Substance Abuse
    1.8. Tic Disorder/Tourette Syndrome
    1.9. Psychotic Disorder
2. **Differential Diagnosis**: **AXIS II Disorder**:
    2.1. Borderline Personality Disorder or Antisocial Personality Disorder
3. **Differential Diagnosis**: **Medications**
    3.1. Mood stabilizers with cognitive dulling side effect
    3.2. Decongestants or beta agonist with psychomotor activation
4. **Differential Diagnosis**: **General Medical Conditions**
    4.1. Hypothyroidism
    4.2. Hypoglycemia
    4.3. Severe anemia
    4.4. Lead poisoning
    4.5. Hearing impairment or vision impairment
    4.6. Sleep disorders
    4.7. Seizure disorders
    4.8. Mental retardation (easy to rule out)
    4.9. Fragile X Syndrome
        4.9.1. Fetal Alcohol Syndrome
        4.9.2. Phenylketonuria
5. **Differential Diagnosis**: **Environmental and other factors**
    5.1. Unsafe or disruptive learning environment
    5.2. School curriculum not well matched to child's ability
    5.3. Family dysfunction or poor parenting

J. Sadek, *A Clinician's Guide to ADHD*,
DOI 10.1007/978-3-319-02359-5_7, © Springer International Publishing Switzerland 2014

5.4. Child abuse or neglect
5.5. Parental psychopathology
5.6. Poor self esteem

- *How to differentiate ADHD from depression*?
  In depression, look for low or irritable mood, suicidal thoughts, plans or intent. Look for loss of interest and pleasure in activities that the person used to enjoy. Look for lack of energy and excessive guilt. Depression is episodic and the person's baseline is different before the episode began.
- *How to differentiate ADHD from Bipolar I Disorder?*
  Bipolar I Disorder could present with Mania or Depression. Mania is episodic. Look for grandiosity, decrease need for sleep, high or irritable mood which is different from the person's baseline, impulsivity in areas that are self damaging, pressured speech that is different than the person's usual speech and look for flight of ideas and racing thoughts. At times, mania would have psychotic symptoms as well. Depression is explained above.
- *How to differentiate ADHD from Generalized Anxiety Disorder (GAD)*?
  GAD would have excessive worry that the person cannot control which extends in many areas. Look for somatic symptoms as tension in muscles, irritability, hyper vigilance, sleep disturbance, lack of energy. Patient may also suffer from panic episodes or other type anxiety disorders as phobia, social anxiety, OCD, PTSD.
- *How to differentiate ADHD from Borderline Personality Disorder (BPD)*?
  In BPD, look for mood fluctuation on hourly basis, significant anger or punching walls, suicidal or parasuicidal behavior or threats, abandonment anxiety, dissociative symptoms or paranoid thoughts and identity disturbance, chronic feelings of emptiness and unstable relationships.
- *How to differentiate ADHD from Antisocial Personality Disorder (ASPS)*?
  In ASPS, look for manipulations, lack of remorse, lack of responsibility, history of Conduct Disorder, consistent irresponsibility, and reckless disregard of safety of self and others.

ADHD Guidelines Available on the Internet

American Psychological Association. http://www.apa.org/topics/adhd/index.aspx
Australian ADHD Draft Guidelines. http://www.nhmrc.gov.au/guidelines/publications/ch54
Canadian ADHD Guidelines. http://www.caddra.ca/cms4/
National Institute for Health and Clinical Excellence (NICE). http://publications.nice.org.uk/attention-deficit-hyperactivity-disorder-cg72
Scottish ADHD Guidelines. http://www.sign.ac.uk/guidelines/fulltext/112/index.html

ADHD Comorbidities

8

8.1 Examples of Comorbidities of ADHD

1. Anxiety Disorder
2. Bipolar Disorder
3. Conduct Disorder
4. Developmental Coordination Disorder
5. Depression
6. Eating Disorder
7. Epilepsy
8. Language and Learning Disorder
9. Obesity
10. Obsessive Compulsive Disorder (OCD)
11. Oppositional Defiant Disorder (ODD)
12. Pervasive Developmental Disorder
13. Sleep Disorder
14. Substance Use Disorder
15. Tic Disorder

8.2 Introduction

High rates of comorbidities with ADHD have been reported in both clinical samples and epidemiological studies. Authors such as Barkley (2002), indicated that comorbidity is generally high in ADHD in both children and adults. Several competing hypothesis are proposed to account for the patterns of comorbidity. Some suggested that maybe one disorder is an early manifestation of the other, development of one disorder increases the risk for the other, one disorder is a subtype of the other (conduct disorder and ADHD may be a subtype of ADHD), the comorbid disorders share common vulnerability factors or genetic and psychosocial factors, each disorder is an expression of phenotypic variability, or finally, each disorder is a separate entity.

J. Sadek, *A Clinician's Guide to ADHD*,
DOI 10.1007/978-3-319-02359-5_8,

8.3 Management of Comorbid Disorders with ADHD

A. **ADHD and Anxiety Disorder**
Around 33 % of children have anxiety as a comorbid disorder with ADHD (MTA Co. 1999). In adults that number could increase to 50 % (Hughes et al. 1999). Treatment of the most disabling condition should be initiated first. Some sources such as CADDRA recommend starting with treating ADHD first. The dose of ADHD medications has to start low and be increased slowly. If anxiety gets worse ADHD medication should be stopped and anti-anxiety medication like SSRI or SNRI can be started.

Atomoxetine has been shown to be effective medication when approaching a patient with anxiety disorder and ADHD (Barkley and Biederman 1997; Connor et al. 2003). Cognitive Behavior Therapy can be used alone for anxiety or in combination with medications. Child and parent training are both useful in CBT for anxiety disorder in children. It is important to inquire about the different types of anxiety as generalized anxiety, panic disorder, phobia, PTSD and social anxiety. It is also important to monitor symptom progression. Mood should also be monitored when treating ADHD with anxiety. Brown mentioned that anxiety may aggravate cognitive deficits seen in ADHD (Brown 2009).

B. **ADHD and Bipolar Disorder (BP)**
Children and adolescents diagnosed with ADHD may also be diagnosed with bipolar disorder (BD) but this comorbid diagnosis is controversial in young children (Wozniak 2005). A sample of patients with ADHD and comorbid Bipolar Disorder were compared to a sample of BP patients with no ADHD. A conclusion has been reached that the ADHD patients with BP were found to have an earlier age of onset of bipolar and short periods of wellness. They also had more irritability, violence, legal problems and less education. That sample had more of mania and depression and more suicide attempts and more comorbidities on Axis I (Birmaher et al. 2010).

Treatment should usually start with managing Bipolar Disorder first and the management is usually more complicated and may require combinations of mood stabilizers and atypical antipsychotics. If patients switch to mania on stimulants (rare), stop the stimulant and start treatment of Biploar Disorder for example using mood stabilizer then go back to a stimulant. Attention should be given to suicide in all age groups and inquiry about substance abuse is important particularly in adolescents. In younger population, parent training and educational accommodation are useful (Consoli et al. 2007; Brown 2009).

C. **ADHD and Conduct Disorder (CD)**
Researchers tried to understand the causes of the high comorbidity between ADHD and conduct disorder (CD) (10–20 % of ADHD patients). They cited several possibilities. One disorder causes another; possibly, one disorder is a risk factor for the development of the other; maybe the disorders share the same related risk factors or there might be a common underlying symptomatic basis for one or more of these behaviors (Mannuzza et al. 2004; Caron and Ruiter 1991).

CD comorbid with ADHD is a severe, persistent condition that has an earlier age at onset and is frequently preceded by ODD, but sometimes ODD can develop in parallel to CD (Biederman et al. 1996; Erhardt and Hinshaw 1994). Co-occurrence of ADHD and CD in adolescents may lead to antisocial behaviors, teen pregnancy, nicotine use, school dropout, substance use or abuse, anxiety or depression and development of antisocial personality disorder as adults (Barkley et al. 2004; Loeber et al. 2002). Parent hostility, low warmth, divorce, and family psychopathology may perpetuate the conduct problems in children and adolescents.

Pharmacotherapy for patients with ADHD, CD and aggression may be useful (stimulant and non-stimulant medication). Combination of medications and psychosocial treatment is beneficial and medications initially should treat the most severe underlying disorder, after which targeting specific symptoms is appropriate (CADDRA 2011).

Conduct problems are generally reduced by all effective ADHD treatments (stimulants and non-stimulant medication and psychosocial treatment (MTA Cooperative Group 2004; Connor et al. 2002). However, the treatment of the ADHD may not be sufficient to resolve all symptoms. It is also important to note that in some cases treatment of ADHD may not improve aggression so monitoring symptoms before and during treatment is important.

Higher doses with a multimodal approach should be attempted, psychosocial treatment, individual behavioral therapy, family interventions and medication optimization, and sometimes, a trial of a mood stabilizer or an atypical antipsychotic may be beneficial (Spencer et al. 2006; Turgay 2005). Group therapy should be avoided in treating conduct disorder.

D. **ADHD and Developmental Coordination Disorder (DCD)**

There might be a shared genetic and familial influence between ADHD and DCD; however, the rate of comorbidity is not clear. DCD may manifest with balance problems, poor handwriting or other manifestations that may be related to cerebellar dysfunction (Barkley 1997). Some authors attempted to examine the benefit of dietary supplementation of fatty acids in DCD but the results were not conclusive (Richardson et al. 2005).

E. **ADHD and Depression**

Evaluating patients for ADHD comorbidities should include the evaluation of mood symptoms and suicide. Lifetime prevalence of depression in youth with ADHD is from 26 to 45 %. Commonly, the onset of ADHD comes first, then anxiety, then depression. Anxious and depressed patients with ADHD respond less to stimulants. Fischer suggested that patients presenting with ADHD and major depressive disorder (MDD) had a higher frequency of generalized anxiety disorder and social phobia and a lower frequency of substance dependence, grade repetition and school suspensions, compared to subjects with ADHD without MDD (Fischer et al. 2007). Many factors contribute to depression including maternal symptoms (Vidair et al. 2011). Moderate to severe depression should be treated first. Untreated ADHD may cause demoralization and anxiety, and in this case, treating ADHD may decrease symptoms of anxiety and depression. Several studies show that a combination of antidepressant and psychostimulant medications are effective. Examples include a combination of Fluoxetine or Paroxetine to stimulants when treating depression or dysthymia with ADHD. Bupropion has shown to be helpful in prominent mood symptoms with ADHD. Older studies showed that Desipramine was helpful in treating depression and ADHD patients. Treatment of depression should be cared for first when there is suicidality, prominent neurovegatative signs, or when depression is the main complaint and ADHD symptoms are mild. Some clinicians find combination of CBT and stimulants very useful in the treatment of mild depression and ADHD.

Clinicians should always keep in mind black box warning of suicide and always assess patients for suicide when indicated (Hechtman 2009; Barkley et al. 2008; www.caddra.ca).

F. **ADHD and Eating disorder**

Kooij in 2004 suggested that Bulemia Nervosa is found to be more prevalent in patients with ADHD versus patients without ADHD (Kooij et al. 2004). Wentz et al. in 2005 found that ADHD is more prevalent in Anorexia Nervosa purging type. Beiderman in 2007 suggested that ADHD females are 3.6 times more likely to meet diagnosis of eating disorders (Biederman et al. 2007). Sobanski et al. in 2007 found that prevalence rate of ADHD in eating disorder is 11.4 %.

G. **ADHD and Epilepsy**

Some studies have suggested a higher rate of symptoms of ADHD in children with epilepsy. The five common epilepsy comorbid conditions are reduced bone health and increased fractures, stroke, depression, migraine, and ADHD (Seindenberg et al. 2009). There is a strong trend toward a higher incidence of epilepsy among children with ADHD than among children without ADHD, and epilepsy in children with ADHD appears to be more severe than in those without (Parisi et al. 2010).

There appears to be a reluctance to diagnose and initiate treatment of ADHD in children with epilepsy (Davis et al. 2010). Older data suggests that stimulant medications could lower seizure threshold, though current data supports the use of stimulants, or Atomoxetine in most cases.

Adult epilepsy patients received relief from sedation with methylphenidate and showed an improved quality of life without significant alteration of seizure control in the presence of antiepileptic medication (Gonzales-Hydrich et al. 2010). New onset seizures can be managed with the addition of an antiepileptic medication (Koneski and Casella 2010).

Some studies suggest that drug interactions between methylphenidate and antiepileptic drugs inhibit metabolism and increase the level of antiepileptics. A conservative approach is still indicated when treating patients with comorbid ADHD and seizure disorder, however, ADHD can be treated in the majority of patients with seizure disorder (CADDRA 2011).

H. **ADHD and Language and Learning Disorder (LD)**

Around one third of individuals with ADHD may fulfill diagnostic criteria for one or more specific learning disorders. ADHD contributes to learning disorders and some aspects of ADHD often overlap with learning disorders. Reading, math and spelling problems are not due to ADHD (Brown 2009).

McGillivray suggested that females with ADHD and LD display more depression than females with ADHD alone, and more than males with ADHD, or ADHD and LD. Presence of learning disorder did not increase anxiety nor aggression in this findings (McGillivray and Baker 2009).

Mathematical learning disorders (MD) are relatively common in school-age children with ADHD and are frequently associated with reading disorders. Having these three comorbid disorders may result in severe impairment (Capano et al. 2008).

Appropriate medication treatment of ADHD symptoms has been shown to improve significant aspects of academic productivity. Medication alone does not establish academic skills that the student has not acquired, but it may help the student's attention to learn. Educational accommodations are required in patients with ADHD and LD (www.caddra.ca).

I. **ADHD and Obesity**

There is a strong association between overweight/obesity and symptoms of ADHD in children, adolescents and adults. It is suggested that the inattentive and impulsive behaviors that characterize ADHD could contribute to overeating. The fast food consumption of foods high in fat, sugar and salt might be contributing factor to obesity in patients with ADHD as a form of self-medication or addiction. This hypothesis can be supported by the finding that addictions are substantially higher among those with ADHD than among the general population. Further research is needed in this area (Davis 2010).

J. **ADHD and OCD**

Some studies suggest that one third of children and adolescents with OCD may have ADHD. Clinicians diagnosing and treating patients for ADHD should routinely enquire about symptoms of OCD. Treatment of both disorders should be carried out simultaneously. There is no indication that treatment of one disorder will improve the symptoms of the other disorder (CADDRA 2011).

Medications used to treat ADHD are not indicated for management of OCD, and medications used for OCD are not effective for treatment of ADHD. Cognitive behavior therapy (CBT) is often an effective treatment of certain types of OCD. CBT treatment with a particular technique of exposure and response prevention has shown to be helpful in management of OCD (Geller 2006; Stein and Lochner 2006; Bolton et al. 1995; Storch et al. 2008).

K. **ADHD and Oppositional Defiant Disorder (ODD)**

Behavioral problems (including ODD, aggression, and delinquency) are highly comorbid with ADHD. Angold et al. in 1999 suggested that ADHD cases are 11 times more likely to have ODD. Between 25 and 65 % of adolescents with ADHD may have concurrent ODD (Spencer et al. 2006). ADHD contributes to ODD, particularly the hyperactive impulsive type (Burns and Walsh 2002). Barkley suggests that parental psychopathology and family stress may lead to disrupted parenting that interacts with child temperament and contributes to ODD. Disrupted parenting may result in the child feeling insecurity, thus responding with a need to control and be defiant.

Persistence of ADHD and ODD in adolescence is linked with an increased risk of delinquent behavior, substance dependence, anxiety, depression, and possibly bipolar disorder.

According to CADDRA, stimulants and Atomoxetine reduce ODD when comorbid with ADHD, but not ODD alone. Treatment requires management of the core symptoms of ADHD plus, in many cases, augmentation with other treatment to address the ODD. Mild cases may respond to behavior management alone, or monotherapy with stimulant medication or Atomoxetine. Moderate to severe cases usually require a combination of pharmacotherapy, which may include alpha2- agonist, and behavior management. Severe or refractory cases may require the introduction of an atypical antipsychotic.

Behavioral therapy for parents and adjunctive parent training in behavioral management methods should be carried out simultaneously. In patients with comorbid ODD with ADHD, it is advisable that the first step is the optimization of pharmacotherapy of ADHD, followed by augmentation with psychosocial treatment, including parenting and other behavioral treatments (Hazell 2010).

L. **ADHD and Pervasive Developmental Disorder (Autism, AS, PDD NOS)**
Some of the most frequent behavioral concerns in PDD are the frequent high rates of activity, impulsivity, and inattention that are often associated with ADHD. Patients who have PDD and ADHD suffer from a severe deficit in social processing, adaptive functioning, and executive control. DSM V considers PDD, an exclusion criteria for ADHD, but this changed in DSM V. Researchers and clinicians have now recognized the importance of attending to both syndromes when both are present and clinically impairing. Up to half of the individuals diagnosed with autism spectrum disorder tend to meet full criteria for ADHD as well. Attentional impairments in autism tend to be more of the "not listening" and "difficulty shifting focus" type than of the "short attention span" and "excessive distractibility" type. Medications used to treat ADHD can help improve ADHD symptoms and impairments in the majority of patients with comorbid ADHD and PDD but the response is considerably lower than typically developed children. Presence of PDD and ADHD make patients at higher risk of experiencing adverse effects, therefore, dosage titration in this population should be done at a slower rate to minimize adverse events (Barkley et al. 1990; Murray 2010; Greenhill et al. 2002; Yoshida and Uchiyama 2004; Keen and Ward 2004; Luteijn et al. 2000; Ehlers and Gillber 1993).

M. **ADHD and Personality Disorders**
Borderline personality disorder (BPD):
ADHD and BPD are known as frequent comorbid disorders. Patients with ADHD have higher lifetime prevalence of BPD than patients without ADH. Philipsen suggested that childhood ADHD may be a risk factor for development of BPD. There are some similarities between the two disorders. They both share deficits in affect regulation, interpersonal functioning, impulse control, and self-esteem. The mechanism of affect regulation, however, differs dramatically in the two conditions. Patients with ADHD may regulate their affect by excessive sports, sexual behavior or impulsive aggressive behavior, while BPD

patients may regulate their affect by dissociation or freezing and finally self-injurious behavior. Some researchers modified Dilectical behavioral therapy (DBT) to fit patients with comorbid ADHD and BPD. Treatment of both disorders can be carried simultaneously (Philipsen 2008; Asherson 2005; Davids and Gastpar 2005; Biederman 2004).

Antisocial Personality disorder (ASPD):

Patients with ADHD have a higher lifetime prevalence of ASPD than patients without ADHD. ASPD is overrepresented in males such that gender appears to have some effect in the disorder. People with ADHD are vulnerable to engage in antisocial behavior and criminal activity for several reasons. First, the high comorbidity with conduct disorder and ASPD. Secondly, by the nature of their cognitive impairment, their offences are more impulsive, not well planned and organized, and they can be more easily caught. Thirdly, they have greater difficulty tolerating the stress of prison life. Treating serious offenders with ADHD may require more complex and comprehensive interventions than non-offending peers. Some authors suggested that diagnosis of ADHD is often missed in incarcerated population. There is a need for early intervention to divert youth away from the criminal trajectory (McKay and Halperin 2001; Young and Thome 2011; Hofvander et al. 2009).

N. ADHD and Sleep Disorder

Periodic limb movement disorder and restless leg syndrome can present with symptoms of ADHD. Snoring and obstructive sleep apnea are associated with neurocognitive symptoms and ADHD in children and adults. Obstructive sleep apnea may contribute to symptoms of ADHD and treatment of sleep problems may have favorable effects on ADHD symptoms. Recent literature suggests that a significant number of children, and more than half of adults, with ADHD reportedly suffer from sleep problems. Some ADHD cases have delayed sleep onset, and in children there might be some bedtime behavioral problems. Middle insomnia might be related to ADHD with anxiety or mood disorder. In ADHD one of the significant findings in some studies was the greater motor activity during sleep. Sleep problems can exacerbate attention problems in school, but it is not clear whether sleep disturbances are intrinsic to ADHD or whether they occur as a result of any underlying primary sleep disorder. There are a significant number of researchers trying to understand and study this area.

It is also important for the clinician to understand if they are treating one disorder as ADHD with sleep problems, or two separate disorders. Some ADHD symptoms were documented in primary sleep disorders so it is important to clarify if the presentation is a comorbidity, or a pure single disorder. Because of the similarity of symptom presentations between ADHD and primary sleep disorders, it has been suggested that misdiagnosis may be occurring between these two disorders.

Stimulant medications may worsen the initial insomnia; some clinicians found that it may improve sleep quality. Treating sleep disorder may improve attention at school, but sleep disorder is not the cause of ADHD, and improved sleep may not translate to better school achievements.

Parents should enforce less stimulating activities at least 1 h or more before bedtime, and restrict television and video games at least 2 h before bedtime. Emphasis on proper sleep hygiene is helpful in both adults and children. Use of Melatonin may improve chronic insomnia in some cases (Guilleminault et al. 1982; Chervin and Archbold 2001; Sowell et al. 2003; Willoughby et al. 2008; Van der Heijden et al. 2007; Mayes et al. 2008; Astill et al. 2012; Youssef et al. 2011; www.caddra.ca).

O. **ADHD and Substance Use Disorder**

Comorbidity of Substance Use disorder and ADHD is high. Literature suggests that one-quarter of adults with SUDs, and one-half of adolescents with SUDs, have ADHD. Adults with SUDs also show a higher risk for ADHD, as well as earlier onset, and more severe SUDs, associated with ADHD. CADDRA guidelines 2011 suggest a higher rate of SUD is recorded in adults with ADHD than in the general population, and ADHD itself is a risk factor for SUD. Patients with conduct or Bipolar disorders co-occurring with ADHD have the greatest likelihood of developing SUD and major comorbidity; ADHD was related to SUDs, but that the main effect was related to conduct disorder.

ADHD can be a significant predictor of early initiation of cigarette smoking; individuals become involved with cigarettes, alcohol, and other drugs of addiction.

Some controversy exists about the relationship between ADHD treatment and substance use. Some researchers suggest that ADHD and SUD-related craving share neurobiological similarities, and that treatment of ADHD may reduce craving for substances and subsequently reduce the risk for relapse to substance use. An aggregate of the literature seems to suggest that early stimulant treatment reduces, or delays, the onset of SUDs and perhaps cigarette smoking into adolescence; however, the protective effect is lost in adulthood.

The self-medication hypothesis is plausible in ADHD. Moreover, the accompanying poor self-judgment and impulsivity associated with ADHD may be conducive to the development of SUD.

Cocaine and stimulant abuse is not overrepresented in ADHD; in fact, marijuana continues to be the most commonly abused agent. Methylphenidate does not have the same abuse liability as cocaine does due to slower dissociation from the site of action, slower uptake into the striatum, and slower binding and dissociation with the dopamine transporter protein relative to cocaine.

Wilens suggested in his review in 2008 that survey studies have indicated that approximately 5 % of college students have misused stimulants. Spencer and his group in 2010 attempted to separate abuse liability among the various extended-release formulations of methylphenidate.

The ADHD group that is at highest risk for diversion and misuses are those with substance abuse and conduct disorder. Both immediate-release, and to a lesser degree extended-release, were diverted or misused. The treatment needs of individuals with SUDs and ADHD need to be considered simultaneously; however, if possible, the SUDs should be addressed initially. If the SUDs are active, immediate attention needs to be paid to stabilization of the addiction.

Depending on the severity and duration of the SUDs, individuals may require inpatient treatment. Self-help groups and CBT can also be helpful. SUD individuals with ADHD require intervention(s) for ADHD (and, if applicable, comorbid psychiatric disorders). Patients with ADHD and SUD require multimodal intervention incorporating both addiction and mental health treatment (Molina and Pelham 2003; Biederman et al. 1995; Faraone and Wilens 2007; Wilens and Upadhyaya 2007; Wilens 2007; Brown 2009; Wilens and Morrison 2011; Wilens et al. 2008; www.caddra.ca).

P. **ADHD and Tic Disorder/Tourette Syndrome (TS)**

The comorbidity of ADHD and Tic disorder is a one-way comorbidity. ADHD is found in 50–75 % of patients with TS, but tics are found in less than 4 % of ADHD patients. Treatment interventions for TS include education about tics and related disorders, clinical monitoring, pharmacological or psychological treatments, and school interventions for children as needed. Some studies indicate that methylphenidate is a safe and effective treatment for ADHD in most children with comorbid tic disorder. In a few cases, stimulants may exacerbate tics, however, mild or episodic tics that are well tolerated by the patient require no treatment.

Atomoxetine, Clonidine, and Guanfacine have shown promise in the management of tics that are comorbid with ADHD. In some cases, use of an antipsychotic medication might be required for the treatment of the disorder (Spencer et al. 1998; Sukhodolsky et al. 2003; Gaffney et al. 2002; Gadow et al. 1999).

References

A 14-month randomized clinical trial of treatment strategies for attention-deficit/hyperactivity disorder. The MTA Cooperative Group. Multimodal Treatment Study of Children with ADHD (1999) Arch Gen Psychiatry 56(12):1073–1086

Angold A et al (1999) Comorbidity. J Child Psychol Psychiatry 49:57–88

Asherson P (2005) Clinical assessment and treatment of attention deficit hyperactivity disorder in adults. Expert Rev Neurother 5(4):525–539

Astill RG, Astill RG, Van der Heijden KB et al (2012) Sleep, cognition, and behavioral problems in school-age children. Psychol Bull 138:1109–1138

Barkley RA (2002) Major life activity and health outcomes associated with attention-deficit/hyperactivity disorder. J Clin Psychiatry 63:10–15

Barkley RA (1997) Attention deficit/hyperactivty. Disorder, self-regulation and time: toward a more comprehensive theory. J Dev Behav Paediatr 18:271–279

Barkley RA et al (2008) ADHD in adults: what the science says. Guilford Press, New York

Barkley RA et al (2004) Young adult follow up of hyperactive children: antisocial activities and drug use. J Child Psychol Psychiatry 45(2):195–211

Barkley RA, Biederman J (1997) Toward a broader definition of the age-of-onset criterion for attention-deficity hyperactity disorder. J Am Acad Child Adolesc Psychiatry 36(9):1204–1210

Barkley RA, DuPaul GJ, McMurray MB (1990) Comprehensive evaluation of attention deficit disorder with and without hyperactivity as defined by research criteria. J Consult Clin Psychol 58(6):775–789

Biederman J (2004) Impact of comorbidity in adults with attention-deficit/hyperactivity disorder. J Clin Psychiatry 65(3):3–7

Biederman J et al (2007) Are girls with ADHD at risk of eating disorders? Results from a controlled, five year prospective study. J Dev Behav Pediatr 28(4):302–307

Biederman J et al (1996) Is childhood oppositional defiant disorder a precursor to adolescent conduct disorder? Findings from a four year follow up study of children with ADHD. J Am Acad Child Adolesc Psychiatry 35(9):1193–1204

Biederman J et al (1995) Psychoactive substance use disorders in adults with attention deficit hyperactivity disorder (ADHD): effects of ADHD and psychiatric comorbidity. Am J Psychiatry 152(11):1652–1658

Birmaher B et al (2010) Psychiatric disorders in preschool offspring of parents with bipolar disorder: the Pittsburgh Offspring Study (BIOS). Am J Psychiatry 167(3):321–330

Bolton D, Luckie M, Steinberg D (1995) Long-term course of obsessive-compulsive disorder treated in adolescence. J Am Acad Child Adolesc Psychiatry 34(11):1441–1450

Brown TE (2009) ADHD comorbidities, 1st edn. American Psychiatric publishing, Washington, DC

Burns GL, Walsh JA (2002) The influence of ADHD on the development of ODD. J Abnorm Child Psychol 30(3):245–256

CADDRA is Candian ADHD Alliance network (2011). www.caddra.ca

Caron C, Ruiter M (1991) Comorbidity in child psychopathology: concepts, issues and research strategies. J Child Psychol Psychiatry 32(7):1063–1080

Capano L, Minden D, Chen SX, Schacher RJ, Ickowicz A (2008) Mathematical learning disorder in school-age children with attention-deficit hyperactivity disorder. Can J Psychiatry 53(6): 392–399

Chervin RD, Archbold KH (2001) Hyperactivity and polysomnographic findings in children evaluated for sleep-disordered breathing. Sleep 24(3):313–320

Connor DF et al (2003) Correlates of comorbid psychopathology in children with ADHD. J Am Acad Child Adolesc Psychiatry 42(2):193–200

Connor DR et al (2002) Psychopharmacology and aggression. A meta-analysis of stimulant effects on over/covert aggression-related behaviors in ADHD. J Am Acad Child Adolesc Psychiatry 41(3):253–261

Consoli A et al (2007) Comorbidity with ADHD decreases response to pharmacotherapy in children and adolescents with acute mania: evidence from meta-analysis. Can J Psychiatry 52(5):3223–3328

Davids E, Gastpar M (2005) Attention deficit hyperactivity disorder and borderline personality disorder. Prog Neuropsychopharmacol Biol Psychiatry 29(6):865–877

Davis C (2010) Attention deficit/hyperactivity disorder: associations with overeating and obesity. Curr Psychiatry Rep 12(5):389–395

Davis SM et al (2010) Epilepsy in children with attention deficit/hyperactivity disorder. Pediatr Neurol 42(5):325–330

Ehlers S, Gillber C (1993) The epidemiology of Asperger syndrome. A total population study. J Child Psychol Psychiatry 34(8):1327–1350

Erhardt and Hinshaw SP (1994) Conduct disorder in childhood: conceptualization, diagnosis, comorbidity, and risk status for antisocial functioning in adulthood. Prog Exp Pers Psychopathol Res pp. 3–44

Faraone S, Wilens TE (2007) Effect of stimulant medications for attention-deficit/hyperactivity disorder on later substance use and the potential for stimulant misuse, abuse and diversion. J Clin Psychiatry 11:15–22

Fischer A et al (2007) The role of comorbid major depressive disorder in the clinical presentation of adult ADHD. J Psychiatr Res 41:991–996

Gadow KD et al (1999) Long-term methylphenidate therapy in children with comorbid attention-deficit hyperactivity disorder and chronic multiple tic disorder. Arch Gen Psychiatry 56(4):330–336

Gaffney GR et al (2002) Risperidone versus clonidine in the treatment of children and adolescents with Tourette's syndrome. J Am Acad Child Adolesc Psychiatry 41(3):330–336

Geller DA (2006) Obsessive-compulsive and spectrum disorders in children and adolescents. Psychiatr Clin N Am 29(2):353–370

Gonzales-Hydrich J et al (2010) Adaptive phase I study of OROS methylphenidate treatment of attention deficit hyperactivity disorder with epilepsy. Epilepsy Behav 18(3):229–237

Greenhill LL et al (2002) Practice parameter for the use of stimulant medications in the treatment of children, adolescents and adults. J Am Acad Child Adolesc Psychiatry 41(2):26S–49S
Guilleminault C et al (1982) Children and nocturnal snoring: evaluation of the effects of sleep related respiratory resistive load and daytime functioning. Eur J Pediatr 139(3):165–171
Hazell P (2010) Review of attention-deficit/hyperactivity disorder comorbid with oppositional defiant disorder. Austr Psychiatry 18(6):556–559
Hechtman L (2009) Comorbidity and neuroimaging in attention-deficit hyperactivity disorder. Can J Psychiatry 54(10):649
Hofvander B, Ossowski D, Lundström S, Anckarsäter H (2009) Continuity of aggressive antisocial behavior from childhood to adulthood: the question of phenotype definition. Int J Law Psychiatry 32(4):224–234
Hughes CW et al (1999) The Texas Children's Medication Algorithm Project: report of the Texas Consensus Conference Panel on Medication Treatment of Childhood Major Depressive Disorder. J Am Acad Child Adolesc Psychiatry 38(11):1442–1454
Keen D, Ward S (2004) Autistic spectrum disorder: a child population profile. Autism 8(1): 39–48
Koneski JA, Casella EB (2010) Attention deficit and hyperactivity disorder in people with epilepsy: diagnosis and implications to treatment. Arq Neuorpsiquiatr 68(1):107–114
Kooij ET et al (2004) Safety of methylphenidate in 45 adults with attention deficit/hyperactivity disorder. A randomized placebo-controlled double blind cross over trial. Psychol Med 34(6):973–982
Loeber R, Burke JD, Lahey BB (2002) What are adolescent antecedents to antisocial personality disorder? Crim Behav Ment Health 12(1):24–36
Luteijn EF et al (2000) How unspecified are disorders of children with a pervasive developmental disorder not otherwise specified? A study of social problems in children with PDD NOS and ADHD. Eur Child Adolesc Psychiatry 9(3):168–179
Mannuzza S et al (2004) Significance of childhood conduct problems to later development of conduct disorder among children with ADHD: a prospective follow up study. J Abnorm Child Psychol 32(5):565–573
Mayes S et al (2008) Non significance of sleep relative to IQ and neuropsychological scores. J Dev Behav Pediatr 29:206–212
McGillivray JA, Baker KL (2009) Effects of comorbid ADHD with learning disabilities on anxiety, depression, and aggression in adults. J Atten Disord 12(6):525–531
McKay KE, Halperin JM (2001) ADHD, aggression, and antisocial behavior across the lifespan. Interactions with neurochemical and cognitive function. Ann New York Acad Sci 931:84–96
Molina BS, Pelham WE Jr (2003) Childhood predictors of adolescent substance use in the longitudinal study of children with ADHD. J Abnorm Psychol 112(3):497–507
Murray MJ (2010) ADHD in the context of autism spectrum disorder. Curr Psychol Rep 12(5):382–388
MTA Cooperative Group (2004) National institute of Mental Health Multimodal Treatment Study of ADHD follow up: changes in effectiveness and growth after the end of treatment. Pediatrics 113(4):762–769
Parisi P et al (2010) Attention deficit hyperactivity disorder in children with epilepsy. Brain Dev 32(1):10–16
Philipsen A (2008) Differential diagnosis and comorbidity of attention-deficit/hyperactivity disorder (ADHD) and borderline personality disorder (BPD) in adults. Eur Arch Psychiatry Clin Neurosci 258(3):192–193
Richardson AJ et al (2005) The Oxford-Durham study. Paediatrics 115:1360
Seindenberg M, Pulsipher DT, Hermann B (2009) Association of epilepsy and comorbid conditions. Future Neurol 4(5):663–668
Sobanski E et al (2007) Psychiatric comorbidity and functional impairment in a clinically referred sample of adults with attention deficit/hyperactivity disorder (ADHD). Eur Arch Psychiatry Clin Neurosci 257(7):371–377
Sowell ER et al (2003) Cortical abnormalities in children and adolescents with attention deficit hyperactivity disorder. Lancet 362(9397):1699–1707

Spencer TJ et al (2006) Efficacy and safety of mixed amphetamine salts extended release (AdderallXR) in the management of oppositional defiant disorder with or without comorbid attention deficit/hyperactivity disorder in school-aged children and adolescents: a 4-week, multicenter, randomized, double-blind, parallel-group, placebo-controlled, forced-dose-escalation study. Clin Ther 28(3):402–418

Spencer T et al (1998) Disentangling the overlap between Tourette's disorder and ADHD. J Child Psychol Psychiatry 39(7):1037–1044

Stein DJ, Lochner C (2006) Obsessive-compulsive spectrum disorders: a multidimensional approach. Psychiatr Clin N Am 29(2):343–351

Storch EA et al (2008) Impact of comorbidity on cognitive-behavioral therapy response in pediatric obsessive-compulsive disorder. J Am Acad Child Adolesc Psychiatry 47(5):583–592

Sukhodolsky DG et al (2003) Disruptive behavior in children with Tourette's syndrome: association with ADHD comorbidity, tic severity, and functional impairment. J Am Acad Child Adolesc Psychiatry 42(1):98–105

Turgay A (2005) Treatment of comorbidity in conduct disorder with attention deficit hyperactivity disorder (ADHD). Essent Psychopharmacol 6(5):277–290

Van der Heijden KB, Smits MG et al (2007) Effect of melatonin on sleep, behavior, and cognition in ADHD and chronic insomnia. J Am Acad Child Adolesc Psychiatry 46:233–241

Vidair HB et al (2011) Screening parents during child evaluation. J Am Acad Child Adolesc Psychiatry 50(5):441–450

Wozniak J (2005) Recognizing and managing bipolar disorder in children. J Clin Psychiatry 66(1):18–23

Wentz E, Lacey JH et al (2005) Neuropsychiatric disorders in adult eating disorder patients. A pilot study. Eur Child Adolesc Psychiatry 14(8):431–437

Wilens TE (2007) The nature of the relationship between attention-deficit/hyperactivity disorder and substance use. J Clin Psychiatry 68(11):4–8

Wilens TE, Morrison NR (2011) The intersection of ADHD and substance abuse. Curr Opin Psychiatry 24(4):280–285, Review

Wilens TE et al (2008) The misuse and diversion of stimulants prescribed for ADHD. J Am Acad Child Adolesc Psychiatry 47:21–31

Wilens TE, Upadhyaya HP (2007) Impact of substance use disorder on ADHD and its treatment. J Clin Psychiatry 68(8):e20

Willoughby MT, Angold A et al (2008) Parent reported ADHD symptomatology and sleep problems in preschool children. J Am Acad Child Adolesc Psychiatry 47:186–194

Yoshida Y, Uchiyama T (2004) The clinical necessity for assessing Attention Deficit/Hyperactivity Disorder (AD/HD) symptoms in children with high-functioning Pervasive Developmental Disorder (PDD). Eur Child Adolesc Psychiatry 13(5):307–314

Young S, Thome J (2011) ADHD and offenders. World J Biol Psychiatry 12(1):124–128

Youssef NA, Ege M et al (2011) Is obstructive sleep apnea associated with ADHD? Ann Clin Psychiatry 23(3):213–224, Review

ADHD Guidelines Available on the Internet

American Psychological Association. http://www.apa.org/topics/adhd/index.aspx

Australian ADHD Draft Guidelines. http://www.nhmrc.gov.au/guidelines/publications/ch54

Canadian ADHD Guidelines. http://www.caddra.ca/cms4/

National Institute for Health and Clinical Excellence (NICE). http://publications.nice.org.uk/attention-deficit-hyperactivity-disorder-cg72

Scottish ADHD Guidelines. http://www.sign.ac.uk/guidelines/fulltext/112/index.html

9 ADHD and Driving

Clinical studies indicate that young drivers with untreated or sub-optimally treated ADHD have between two to four time as many Motor Vehicle Collisions (MVC) and moving violations than a comparable non-ADHD population. These morbidities are seen independent of comorbidity. The problem profile commonly indicates Driving Anger or Road Rage. The presence of comorbid substance use disorders and ADHD significantly magnifies problem driving risks. There is a continuum of neurodevelopmental immaturities in executive control accompanied by lack of driving experience in many young drivers that underlie deficient cognitive processes related to problems with attention, impulse control and emotional regulation leading to problem driving styles. These neurodevelopmental compromises are more pronounced in ADHD populations.

Based on simulator studies, stimulant medication may reduce cognitive difficulties related to ADHD problem driving. However, on the road real time demonstrating the benefit of stimulants is limited. Compliance with stimulant medication is poor, particularly at time of maximal driving risk for young drivers. Practical restrictions on cell phone use, night time and weekend driving and use of manual transmission may all have an impact on improving driving performance. Psychosocial and legislative measure may prove to be a more effective preventative public health measure in the long run. Current CMA Guidelines require clinicians to be aware that if ADHD drivers have a demonstrated problem with driving and are non-compliant with treatment they have a duty to report their concerns to the Provincial Ministries of Transportation. Reporting in Alberta, Quebec and Nova Scotia is discretionary.

Discussion with young drivers and their families should include a discussion of functional impairment in the real world. It may have utility in developing clinical contracts with young drivers and their families for compliance with medications and school performance in exchange for access to a motor vehicle. Documentation

This entire chapter is an excerpt of an article by Dr. Laurence Jerome, MD, FRCPC, and has been reproduced with permission.

J. Sadek, *A Clinician's Guide to ADHD*,
DOI 10.1007/978-3-319-02359-5_9,

of discussions regarding driving safety along with the use of an assessment of driving style and behavior would demonstrate that the clinician is exercising due diligence for their ADHD patients around driving safety issues.

9.1 Epidemiology of ADHD and Problem Driving

Canadian psychiatrists, Tillmand and Hobbs in 1949, hold the distinction of publishing the first article on psychiatric illness and problem driving. The first observation on the link between ADHD in childhood and later problem driving comes from the early observations in Montreal by Gabrielle Weiss and Lily Hechtman (1984) who showed an increase prevalence of problem driving in a cohort of ADHD patients diagnosed in childhood followed up to their adult years. Since then an emerging body of literature both from clinical samples and epidemiological cohorts has demonstrated an increased prevalence of both MVC's and moving violations in driver with ADHD. Recent findings from a large longitudinal prospective cohort study of functional outcomes in Adult ADHD from clinical and community samples illustrate similar adult outcomes for problem driving as part of the profile of adult functional impairment (Barkley et al. 2009). ADHD is now a recognized predisposing factor to Traumatic Brain Injury secondary to MVC (Levin et al. 2007). These findings should be seen within the larger context of an escalating incidence of mortality and chronic morbidity costs from driving amongst all drivers world-wide (World Health Organization 2004). Two meta-analyses suggest that ADHD populations are three times more likely to suffer injury and four times more likely to be involved in collisions, and up to five times as likely to speed. Published studies have involved combined type ADHD syndromes with no data on subtypes or symptom clusters (Truls 2003; Jerome et al. 2006). Unpublished clinical case material from this reviewers' Adult ADHD practice contains a small sample of cases of inattentive ADHD without impulsiveness referred for problems with attention causing problem driving. Unlike the normal population the improvement in driving with age and experience may not happen with older ADHD patients who report similar prevalence of problem driving events as younger drivers. Also male and female ADHD drivers appear to be at similar driving outcomes (Cox and Coleman 2009). Teenage drivers with attention problems drive significantly more often than other teenage drivers (Woodward et al. 2000); hence negative driving outcomes for this high risk population for problem driving is compounded by an increased exposure risk.

Whilst many studies implicate associated comorbidities such as conduct disorder and emotional disorder, as well as substance use disorder as accounting for a significant amount of the increased prevalence of problem driving, the longitudinal studies have been able to demonstrate an independent risk factor for ADHD, separate from comorbid illness (Woodward et al. 2000; Nada-Raja et al. 1997). Problems with Driving Anger or Road Rage are commonly seen in problem drivers and ADHD independent of comorbidities (Richards et al. 2002; Malta et al. 2005). Experimental research suggests that the driving of a sober adult with ADHD is comparable to a typical adult with .08 blood alcohol level (Weafer et al. 2008).

Recent studies have demonstrated that the ADD influences on problem driving outcomes are made "differentially worse" in the presence of comorbidities such as alcoholism (Barkley et al. 2009; Levin et al. 2007).

9.2 Neurodevelopmental Basis for Problem Driving in Adults with ADHD

Emerging data on adolescent brain development argue for the primacy of executive functioning deficits in explaining proneness for risk-taking behaviors and a range of physical accidents in young adults. Abundant empirical evidence shows that age-related brain changes are regional in nature (Sowell et al. 2004; Blakemore and Choudbury 2006). The frontal lobe, including the prefrontal cortex (PFC) Shaw and colleagues have recently demonstrated significantly increased delay in maturation of key anatomical areas in those brain regions associated with the development of executive function in ADHD children and adolescents in comparison to age and sex matched controls (Shaw et al. 2007). Recent conceptual models of ADHD have characterized the condition as being mediated by deficits in executive function control (Barkley 1997). Core functional impairments in executive function related to response inhibition, working memory and flexible strategic response help to explain both general ADHD pathology and its specific manifestations in problem driving. Whilst lack of driving experience may be a general factor leading to increased accident risk in young adults, the neurobiological basis of immature executive functioning present in young adults, in general, and in ADHD populations in particular who manifest ongoing immaturieis in adaptive function is thought to be paramount (Jerome and Segal 2005). This maturational deficit of social and cognitive delay, typically observable from early childhood and continuing through the early adult years, would help explain the particularly acute driving vulnerability in young adults with ADHD (Stein et al. 1995). As Barkley et al. (1996, 2002) has noted it was not the knowledge base of driving skills that differentiated the driving problems in ADHD youth so much as their inability to apply these rules at the appropriate time and under the appropriate circumstances.

9.3 Effects of Medication on Improving Driving Performance in ADHD Drivers

Experimental studies indicate that stimulants and to a lesser extent non-stimulant drugs used to treat ADHD improve areas of driving performance. Since young drivers are at increased risk driving later in the night when immediate release stimulants appear to be ineffective, the long acting medications have evident advantages. Most of the evidence for the beneficial effects of stimulant medication comes from simulator studies with a very limited number of reports of benefit based on actual driving on the road. Currently there are 10 published studies; 8 with methylphenidate mostly immediate release approximately 290 subjects in all (Jerome et al. 2006; Cox and Coleman 2009; Cox et al. 2008; Kay et al. 2009). Currently, the benefit of

Atomoxetine on subjective driver report lacks support from more objective simulator findings. At the time of writing (May, 2010), there are no studies examining Lisdexamfetamine. A significant limitation of these studies are that they are all industry funded. They generally involve a fixed dose protocol so medication dosages for individual subject were not optimized. Effects sizes from methylphenidate improved simulator performance vary from 0.4 to 1.8. The biggest effect sizes are seen in samples of young drivers in their late teens and early twenties on extended release preparations. Two further studies utilizing a randomized cross-over designed with optimized stimulant dosing in real driving situations have shown positive results on driving with methylphenidate (Cox et al. 2009; Verster et al. 2008).

The medications likely mediate their effect via improvement in executive functioning particularly on tasks of complex attention as well as response inhibition (Jerome and Segal 2000). One open label study of on the road driving over an extended period of 12 months suggests that problem driving is responsive to trials of stimulants as measured by self and collateral reported driving style (Jerome and Segal 2001). Short duration of action and poor long term compliance with medication use remains a significant problem particularly at the time of maximum vulnerability, evenings, weekends and school vacations (Marcus et al. 2005). The question of rebound, even in long acting stimulants, remains a potential theoretical problem (Cox and Coleman 2009).

9.4 Future Research: Psychosocial and Behavioral Interventions

The requirement of graduated licensing and psychosocial family based contracting with at-risk adolescent drivers, offers hope of useful behavioral change (Fabiano GA et al., A feasibility study of a parent and teen behavioral intervention targeting safe driving for teens with ADHD, personal communication, 2009, Unpublished). Legislated interventions within the internal environment of the vehicle that regulate the use of cell phones, govern speed and also provide appropriate cues to the distracted driver may prove to be a more effective intervention for improving road safety than individual treatment regimens given the emerging evidence of the lack of voluntary use of optional in-car speed governors in drivers prone to speeding (Jamson 2006). Further research focused on the effect of motivational interviewing on compliance, and the effect of combining psychosocial treatment with pharmacological treatment on driving performance and road safety will be helpful.

9.5 Medicolegal Reporting Requirements and the Individual Clinician

Canadian rules to determining medical fitness to operate motor vehicles are moving in the direction of requiring physicians to report ADHD drivers to the Ministry of Transportation who, in their own clinical judgment, have demonstrated problem driving secondary to poorly controlled ADHD symptoms (Canadian Medical

Association 2006). This initiative was started in 2006. Clinical assessment may be assisted by using a standardized tool to help guide them in evaluating patient driving risk and the response to treatment (Jerome and Segal 2005). Available instruments includes Jerome Driving Questionnaire which is free from www.caddra.ca.

References

Barkely RA (2006) Effects of two doses of alcohol on simulator driving performance in adults with attention-deficit hyperactivity disorder. Neuropsychology 20:77–87

Barkley RA (1997) ADHD and the nature of self-control. Guilford Press, New York

Barkley RA, Murphy KR, Kwasnik D (1996) Motor vehicle driving competencies and risks in teens and young adults with attention deficit hyperactivity disorder. Pediatrics 98(6): 1089–1095

Barkley RA, Murphy KR, DuPaul GJ, Bush T (2002) Driving in young adults with attention-deficit/hyperactivity disorder: knowledge, performance, adverse outcomes, and the role of executive functioning. J Int Neuropsychol Soc 8:655–672

Barkley RA, Murphy KR, Fischer M (2009) ADHD in adults: what the science says. Guildford Press, New York

Blakemore SJ, Choudbury S (2006) Development of the adolescent brain: implications for executive function and social cognition. J Child Psychol Psychiatry 47(3–4):296–312

Canadian Medical Association (2006) Determining medical fitness to operate motor vehicles. CMA driver's guide, 7th edn. The Association, Ottawa

Cox DJ, Coleman MT (2009) Attention deficit/hyperactivity disorder (ADHD) and driving safety. In: Verster JE, Pandi-Perumal SR, Ramaekers JG, de Glier JJ (eds) Drugs, driving and traffic safety. Birkhii user Verlag, Switzerland, pp 315–330

Cox DJ, Mikami A, Cox BS, Coleman MT, Mahmood A, Sood A, Moore M, Burket R, Murkel RL (2008) Effect of long-acting OROS methylphenidate on routine driving in young adults with attention-deficit/hyperactivity disorder. Arch Pediatr Adolesc Med 162:793–794

Cox DJ, Davis M, Ibia A, Burket R, Merkel RL (2009) Driving Safety in Young Adults diagnosed with Attention Deficit Hyperactivity Disorder (ADHD) with and without long acting transdermal methylphenidate therapy (Daytrana). In: Poster presentation. American Psychiatric Association

DSM-5: options being considered for the diagnosis of Adult ADHD. 2 Feb 2010. 2010 American Psychiatric Association. http://www.dsm5.org/Proposed%20Revision%20Attachments/APA%20Options%20for%20ADHD.pdf. Accessed 26 Apr 2010

Jamson S (2006) Would those who need it use it? Investigating the relationship between drivers speed choice and their use of a voluntary ISA system. Transport Res F 9:195–206

Jerome L, Segal AU (2000) ADHD and executive function and problem driving. ADHD Rep 8(2):7–11

Jerome L, Segal AU (2001) Benefit of long term stimulants on driving in adults with ADHD. J Nerv Ment Dis 189(1):63–64

Jerome L, Segal AU (2005) Prediction of driving accident risk in novice drivers in Ontario: the development of a screening instrument. In: International conference on driver behavior and training (2nd 2005 Edinburgh, Scotland), Driver behavior and training, vol 2 – (Human factors in road and rail transport), Editor Lisa Dorn, pp 207–222

Jerome L, Segal A (2005) Validation of a driving Questionnaire for patients with ADHD: the Jerome Driving Questionnaire (JDQ). J Am Acad Child Adolesc Psychiatry (1):151

Jerome L, Segal A, Habinkski L (2006) What we know about ADHD and driving risk: a literature review meta-analysis and critique. J Can Acad Child Adolesc Psychiatry 15(3):105–125

Kay GG, Michaels A, Pakull B (2009) Simulated driving changes in young adults with ADHD receiving mixed amphetamine salts extended release and atomoxetine. J Atten Disord 12:316–329

Levin H, Hanten G, Max J, Li X, Swank P, Ewing-Cobbs L, Dennis M, Menefee DS, Schachar R (2007) Symptoms of attention-deficit/hyperactivity disorder. J Dev Behav Pediatr 28:108–118
Malta LS, Blanchard EB, Freidenberg BM (2005) Psychiatric and behavioral problems in aggressive drivers. Behav Res Ther 43:1467–1484
Marcus SC, Wan GJ, Kemner JE, Olfson M (2005) Continuity of methylphenidate treatment for attention-deficit/hyperactivity disorder. Arch Pediatr Adolesc Med 159:572–578
Nada-Raja S, Landley JO, McGee R, Williams SM, Begg DJ, Reeder AI (1997) Inattentive and hyperactive behaviors and driving offenses in adolescence. J Am Acad Child Adolesc Psychiatry 36:515–522
Reimer B, Mehler B, D'Ambrosio LA, Fried R (2010) The impact of distractions on young adult drivers with attention deficit hyperactivity disorder (ADHD). Accid Anal Prev 42:842–851
Richards TL, Deffenbacher JL, Rosen LA (2002) Driving anger and other driving –related behaviors in high and low ADHD symptom college students. J Atten Disord 6(1):25–38
Shaw P et al (2007) ADHD is characterized by a delay in cortical maturation. Proc Natl Acad Sci 104:19649–19654
Sowell ER, Thompson PM, Leonard CM, Welcome SE, Tan E (2004) Longitudinal mapping of cortical thickness and brain growth in normal children. J Neurosci 24(38):8223–8231
Stein MA, Szumowski E, Blondis TA, Roizen NJ (1995) Adaptive skills dysfunction in ADD and ADHD children. J Child Psychol Psychiatry 36:663–670
Tillman WA, Hobbs GE (1949) The accident-prone automobile driver. Am J Psychiatry 106:321–331
Truls V (2003) Impairment, diseases, and their relative risks of accident involvement: results from meta analysis. Impaired Motorists, Methods of Roadside Testing and Assessment of Licensing (IMMORTAL). Deliverable R1.1. From: http://www.immortal.or.at/index/php. Retrieved 1 Nov 2005
Verster JC, Bekker EM, de Roos M, Minova A, Eijken EJ, Kooij JJ, Buitelaar JK, Kenemans JL, Verbaten MN, Olivier B, Volkerts ER (2008) Methylphenidate significantly improves driving performance of adults with attention-deficit hyperactivity disorder: a randomized crossover trial. J Psychopharmacol 22(3):230–237
Weafer J, Camarillo D, Fillmore MT, Milich R, Marczinski CA (2008) Simulated driving performance of adults with ADHD: comparisons with alcohol intoxication. Exp Clin Psychopharmacol 16:251–263
Weiss G, Hechtman L, Perlman T (1984) Hyperactives as young adults: past and current substance abuse and antisocial behavior. Am J Orthopsychiatry 54(3):415–425
Woodward LJ, Fergusson DM, Horwood LJ (2000) Driving outcomes of young people with attentional difficulties in adolescence. J Am Acad Child Adolesc Psychiatry 39(5):627–634
World Health Organization (2004) World report on road traffic injury prevention. WHO, Geneva

10 Pharmacological Management of ADHD

10.1 Introduction

Australian Draft Guidelines Recommendations
(Please see copyright permission page at the beginning of this book.)

> Medications should only be used when symptoms are pervasive across settings (e.g., school and home), and are causing significant impairment in academic, social or behavioral function, and after careful consideration of non-pharmacological approaches.

10.2 General Recommendations

A multimodal approach is advocated for treatment of ADHD. Pharmacological treatment should be part of a comprehensive management plan that includes psychosocial treatment and education or vocational interventions.

Clinical practice is not always consistent with the indication stated in the product monograph. Clinicians are encouraged to know the product monograph recommendations, guidelines and expert recommendations.

Clinicians should discuss with their patient and the family (as appropriate) the indications for using the medication, the adverse side effects and their management, risk and benefit of treatment, alternative therapies, and any other information that

---

Warning This document does not include all of the medications, safety, and efficacy information available. It is provided as a professional courtesy to provide pertinent data that will assist you in forming your own conclusions and making your own decisions. Please consult each Product Monograph of each product for detailed prescribing information.

J. Sadek, *A Clinician's Guide to ADHD*,
DOI 10.1007/978-3-319-02359-5_10, © Springer International Publishing Switzerland 2014

would help the patient before obtaining consent for treatment. Clearly defined goals should be identified prior to commencing a trial of medication treatment.

Cost should be considered particularly when the patient has no medication coverage.

Family history of response and patient's prior early response to ADHD medications should be obtained. It can guide the clinician in their decision to select a medication.

Comorbid psychiatric or medical condition and current medications, and over the counter products may also influence the selection of ADHD medication treatment.

When psychostimulant treatment is used, it should be continued for as long as it is of assistance to the person with ADHD and is not causing unacceptable side effects.

In school age children, adolescents and adults, Methylphenidate (MPH), or amphetamine-based products should be used as a first line pharmacological treatment. Atomoxetine can be used as a first line in certain situations highlighted in the table below.

Extended release formulation has the advantage of avoiding multiple dosing, and the stigma of taking medications during school for students.

In some cases the combined use of immediate release and extended release forms is required. This should only be considered if there is inadequate symptom control with the extended release form.

10.3 Stimulant Medication

10.3.1 General Information About Stimulant Medications

Stimulants (either methylphenidate or amphetamine) are the most effective drug treatment for ADHD, with large effect sizes of about 1 when using rating scales in randomized controlled trials (Pliszka 2007; Prince 2006). Methylphenidate and mixed amphetamine salts are considered comparable in efficacy; 65–75 % of children, adolescents, and adults achieved therapeutic response compared with 4–30 % taking placebo in controlled studies (Pliszka 2007; Prince 2006). When one stimulant is ineffective, there is a 20–40 % chance that the other stimulant will be effective, and it should be tried. When both methylphenidate and amphetamine salts have been tried, stimulant response rates are as high as 85 % (Pliszka 2007).

The following table explains the different options in ADHD treatment. The dosage recommendations are based on Product Monographs, but clinicians may consider the expert recommendations as what is available at www.caddra.ca. Please refer to this link for further information http://www.caddra.ca/cms4/pdfs/Medication_Chart_English_CANADA.pdf.

10.4 Stimulants

Methylphenidate-based products		Amphetamine-based products	
MPHIR (Ritalin*) 10 and 20 mg tablets	Start with 5–10 mg b.i.d. to t i d. Increase by 5–10 mg weekly Maximum dose 60 mg for children and adolescents and 60 mg for adults (some experts recommend higher doses)	**Dexedrine*** (Dextroamphetamine) 5 mg tablet	Start with 2.5–5 mg b.i.d. Increase by 5 mg weekly Maximum dose 40 mg for children, adolescents and adults
Ritalin* SR (MPH) 20 mg tablet	Start with 20 mg in the morning Increase by 20 mg weekly **Maximum** dose 60 mg for children and for adolescents and adults 60 mg (some experts recommend higher doses)	**Dexedrin* Spansule*** 10 and 15 mg spansule	Start with 10 mg in the morning Increase by 5–10 mg weekly Maximum dose 40 mg for all ages
Biphentin* 10, 15, 20, 30, 40, 50, 60, 70, 80 mg capsule **(1st line)**	Start with 10–20 mg in the morning Increase by 10 mg weekly Maximum dose 60 mg for children and 80 mg for adolescents and adults *40 % immediate and 60 % delayed release*	**Adderall XR*** (Amphetamine mixed salt) 5, 10, 15, 20, 25, 30 mg capsules **(1st line)** *Delivers 50 % immediate and 50 % delayed release*	Start with 5–10 mg in the morning for children, 10 mg for adolescents and adults Increase by 5–10 mg weekly Maximum dose 30 mg for children and 30 mg for adolescents and adults
Concerta* 18, 27, 36, 54 mg tablets **(1st line)**	Start with 18 mg in the morning Increase by 18 mg weekly Maximum dose 54 mg for children, 54 mg for adolescents, and 72 mg for adults	**Vyyanse*** (Lisdexamfetamin dimeyslate) 20, 30, 40, 50, 60 mg capsules **(1st line)**	Start with 20–30 mg in the morning Increase by 10 mg weekly Maximum dose 60 mg for children and 70 mg for adolescents and adults
MPH ER-C 18, 27, 36, 54 mg tablet	Start with 18 mg in the morning Increase by 18 mg weekly Maximum dose 54 mg for all ages according to product monograph		

*trade name in Canada

10.4.1 Additional Information About Medications (Alphabetical Order) – Stimulants

Adderall XR® (Mixed Amphetamine Salts) (Source: CADDRA2011)

Adderall XR® is a controlled substance made up of a combination of different amphetamine salts that have effects on the noradrenaline and dopamine neurotransmitters. The mixed amphetamine salts in this medication are: Dextroamphetamine sulfate, dextro-, levoapmphetamine sulfate, dextro-, levoamphetamine aspartate, and dextroamphetamine saccharate. Adderall consists of 25 % levo- and 75 % dextroamphetamine in four salts. It is used in the treatment of ADHD. The capsules can be opened and the beads inside the capsule can be sprinkled with no loss in efficacy. Adderall XR is a capsule with at 50:50 ratio of immediate to delayed release beads designed to release drug content in a long acting time course. Adderall XR administered in once daily doses of 20, 40 or 60 mg appears to be safe and efficacious for treating adults with ADHD. The treatment response rate and side effect profile of methylphenidate-based versus amphetamine-based products are similar.

Biphentin® (Source: CADDRA)

Biphentin® is a controlled release methylphenidate (MPH) product and uses a multilayer release (MLRTM) delivery system that is long acting and produces 40 % immediate and 60 % delayed release. It can be opened and sprinkled on food, making it useful for children who cannot swallow pills, and since the beads within each capsule are all the same, there is no concern of pharmacokinetics problem in the body when it is poured. Patients can be switched from MPH easily (switching conversion rate: 10 mg t.i.d. MPH=30 mg Biphentin). In a study by Schachar et al. (2008), Biphentin was given once daily and produced equivalent improvements in behavioral and cognitive measures, and had a duration of effect at least as long as that of immediate release MPH give twice given twice daily (Fig. 10.1).

Concerta®

The information contained below is direct from manufacturer, Janssen Ltd. (with permission) and does not include all of the Concerta® safety and efficacy information available. Please consult Concerta® Product Monograph for detailed prescribing information. Permission for reproduction has been received.

<u>Product Summary</u>

Concerta® (methylphenidate HCI) is indicated for the treatment of Attention Deficit Hyperactivty Disorder (ADHD) in children (6–12 years of age), adolescents (13–18 years of age) and adults (>18 years of age).

Concerta® should not be taken by children under 6 years of age.

There is no data available for the use of Concerta® in patients over 65 years of age.

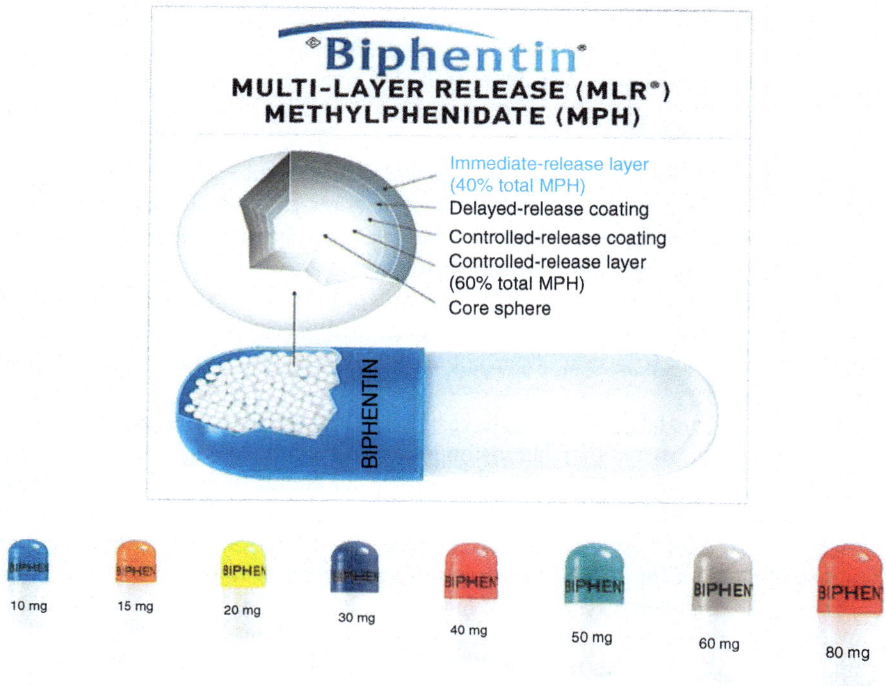

Fig. 10.1 Image copyright permission obtained – Purdue Pharma

Concerta® is indicated as an integral part of a total treatment program for ADHD that may include other measures (psychological, educational, social). Effectiveness more than 4 weeks in children and adolescents, and for more than 7 weeks in adults has not been systematically evaluated in placebo-controlled trials. Physicians electing to use Concerta® for extended periods should periodically re-evaluate the long term usefulness of the drug for the individual patient.

<u>Warnings and Precautions</u>

Theoretically, there exists a pharmacological potential for all ADHD drugs to increase the risk of sudden/cardiac death. Although confirmation of an incremental risk for sudden/cardiac death arising from treatment with ADHD medications is lacking, prescribers should consider this potential risk, and Concerta® generally should not be used in patients with known structural cardiac abnormalities, cardiomyopathy, serious heart rhythm abnormalities, coronary artery disease or other serious cardiac problems.

Prior to initiating sympathomimetic treatments, a personal and family history and physical exam should be obtained to assess for cardiac disease. In patients with relevant risk factors, further cardiovascular evaluation may be considered (e.g., electrocardiogram and echocardiogram), based on the clinician's judgment. Patients who develop symptoms suggestive of cardiac disease during ADHD treatment should undergo a prompt cardiac evaluation.

Concerta® should be given cautiously to patients with a history of drug dependence or alcoholism. Chronic abusive use can lead to marked tolerance and psychological dependence with varying degrees of abnormal behavior.

Concerta® should not be used in patient with pre-existing gastrointestinal narrowing.

There is some clinical evidence that methylphenidate may lower the convulsive threshold in patients with a prior history of seizures, in patients with prior EEG abnormalities in the absence of seizures, and, very rarely, in the absence of history of seizures and no prior EEG evidence of seizures.

Stimulants may impair the ability of the patient to operate potentially hazardous machinery or vehicles. Patients should be cautioned accordingly until they are reasonably certain that Concerta® does not adversely affect their ability to engage in such activities.

Symptoms of visual disturbances have been encountered in rare cases. Difficulties with accommodation and blurring vision have been reported.

Administration of stimulants may exacerbate symptoms of behavior disturbance and thought disorder in patients with a pre-existing psychotic disorder. Stimulants should be used with care to treat ADHD in patients with comorbid bipolar disorder because of concern for possible induction of a mixed/manic episode.

Treatment-emergent psychotic or manic symptoms, e.g., hallucinations, delusional thinking or mania in children and adolescents without a prior history of psychotic illness or mania can be caused by stimulants at usual doses. Although there is no systematic evidence that stimulants cause aggressive behavior or hostility, these are often observed in children and adolescents with ADHD and have been reported in clinical trials and the postmarketing experience of some medications indicated for the treatment of ADHD.

Adverse Events

The most common adverse events reported in children treated with Concerta®, regardless of causality, were: headache (95), upper respiratory tract infections (8 %), abdominal pain (7 %), vomiting, anorexia, insomnia, cough increased and pharyngitis (4 % each).

The most common adverse event reported in adolescents treated with Concerta®, regardless of causality, were: headache (9 %), accidental injury (6 %), insomnia (4 %), fever, vomiting and rhinitis (3 %).

The most common adverse events reported in adults treated with Concerta®, regardless of causality, were: decreased appetite (20–34 %), headache (17–26 %), dry mouth (7–21 %), insomnia (12–17 %), and nausea (8–16 %).

Drug Interactions

Alcohol may exacerbate the CNS adverse effect of psychoactive drugs. Therefore, patients undergoing Concerta® therapy should be advised to avoid alcohol during treatment.

Because of possible increases in blood pressure and heart rate, Concerta® should be used cautiously with drugs with similar pharmacological actions.

Human pharmacologic studies have shown that methlyphenidate may inhibit the metabolism of courmarin anticoagulants (e.g., warfarin), anticonvulsants (e.g., phenobarbital, phenytoin, primidone) and some antidepressants (tricyclics and selective serotonin reuptake inhibitors). Downward dose adjustment of these drugs may be required when given concomitantly with methylphenidate.

Concerta® is contraindicated during treatment with monoamine oxidase inhibitors, and also within a minimum of 14 days following discontinuation of a monoamine oxidase inhibitor (hypertensive crises may result).

Dosage and Administration

Concerta® tablets must be swallowed whole with liquids, and must not be chewed, divided or crushed.

The tablet shell, along with insoluble core components, is eliminated from the body; patients should not be concerned if they occasionally notice something that looks like a tablet in their stool.

The recommended starting dose of Concerta® for patients who are not currently taking methylphenidate, or for patients who are on stimulants other than methylphenidate, is 18 mg once daily for all age groups. The maximum dosage for children and adolescents (6–18 years of age) is 54 mg once per day and 72 mg once per day for adults (>18 years of age).

Reference

1. Concerta® (methylphenidate hydrochloride) extended-release tablets Product Monograph.

Dexedrine® and Dexedrine® Spansules (DEX)

Dextroamphetamine (DEX) is classified as a psychostimulant which exact mechanism of action is not fully known but it is suggested that it blocks the re-uptake of dopamine and norepinephrine, binds the dopamine transporter protein, and increases the release of dopamine making dopamine more available in the presynaptic neuron. That may explain its increased potency over MPH (i.e., only half the dose is required). Dexedrine® Spansules last about 6–8 h (Kolar 2008). The drug has been available in Canada for decades.

DEX immediate release has a short half-life of 4–6 h, and requires multiple dosing of two to three times a day. DEX is quickly absorbed after oral administration and half the dose is eliminated unchanged and the other half goes through extensive metabolism mostly to benzoic acid. DEX can be used to supplement the long acting medications if needed or when more flexibility in dosing is required (Kolar 2008; CADDRA 2011).

Methylphenidate (MPH) Ritalin®, Ritalin® SR and Generic Products

MPH is classified as a psychostimulant and is a controlled substance which exact mechanism of action is not fully known, but it is suggested that it blocks the re-uptake of dopamine and norepinephrine, and binds the dopamine transporter protein. The efficacy and safety of MPH has been well established for decades with significant reduction in the core ADHD symptoms. MPH is rapidly and extensively absorbed after oral administration. After absorption, it undergoes significant first pass metabolism in the liver by hydrolysis and 80 % of the drug is excreted as

Ritalinic acid (Kolar 2008; Connor 2005). MPH can be dissolved and injected. That can create some abuse potential, but remains much less that cocaine. Currently there are three pharmaceutical formulations of MPH: immediate release (IR), sustained release, and long acting. Ritalin® SR which is an intermediate acting sustained release formulation but produces variable results due to pharmacokinetic changes, so its use is less useful. An immediate release or short acting preparation can be used as a supplement to the long acting preparation or when flexibility in dosing is required.

Vyvanse®

The information contained below is direct from manufacturer, Shire PLC, (with permission) and does not include all of the Vyvanse® safety and efficacy information available. Please consult Vyvanse® Product Monograph for detailed prescribing information.

Product Summary

VYVANSE® (lisdexamfetamine dimesylate capsules) is indicated for the treatment of Attention Deficit Hyperactivity Disorder (ADHD). VYVANSE® is indicated as an integral part of a total treatment program for ADHD that may include other measures (psychological, educational/vocational, and social) for patients with this syndrome (VYVANSE® Product Monograph).

VYVANSE® is a prodrug of D-amphetamine. A prodrug is an inactive compound that must undergo chemical or enzymatic transformation to an active form prior to exhibiting a pharmacological response (Stanczak 2006).

After oral administration, LDX is rapidly absorbed from the GI tract and converted to D-amphetamine, which is responsible for the drug's activity, and L-lysine by hydrolysis in the blood (VYVANSE® Product Monograph). It was believed that conversion of LDX occurred by first pass intestinal and/or hepatic metabolism. However, recent preclinical studies suggest that LDX is absorbed intact in the small intestine into the portal circulation and that the enzymatic hydrolysis of LDX to D-amphetamine occurs primarily in the blood by red blood cells, with a smaller amount converted in the gastrointestinal tract (Pennick 2010).

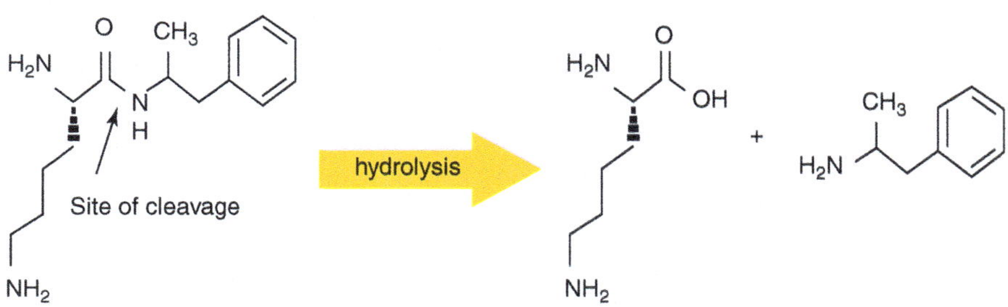

Lisdexamfetamine dimesylate* (Prodrug) — *l*-lysine — *d*-amphetamine (Active Drug)

The mode of therapeutic action of amphetamine in ADHD is not known (Vyvanse® Product Monograph). Amphetamines are thought to block the reuptake of norepinephrine and dopamine into the presynaptic neuron and increase the release of these monoamines into the extraneuronal space (Pliszka 2001). Unlike amphetamine, the parent drug, lisdexamfetamine, does not bind to the sites responsible for the reuptake of norepinephrine and dopamine in vitro (Vyvanse® Product Monograph).

In patients who are either starting treatment for the first time or switching from another medication, 30 mg once daily in the morning is the usual starting dose. When in the judgement of the clinician a lower dose is appropriate, patients may begin treatment with 20 mg once daily in the morning. In clinical studies, doses of 20–70 mg/day were shown to be effective, although no additional benefit was demonstrated at doses greater than 30 mg/day, and adverse events and discontinuations were more frequent at higher doses. Doses greater than 70 mg/day of Vyvanse® have not been studied. If the physician, based on clinical judgment, decides a dose increase is warranted for an individual patient, the maximum dose should not exceed 60 mg/day; dosage may be adjusted at approximately weekly intervals (Vyvanse® Product Monograph).

Vyvanse® may be taken with or without food. Vyvanse® capsules may be taken whole, or the capsule may be opened and the entire contents dissolved in a glass of water. If the patient is using the solution administration method, the solution should be consumed immediately; it should not be stored. The dose of a single capsule should not be divided (Vyvanse® Product Monograph).

Vyvanse® is contraindicated in patients with Advanced arteriosclerosis, Symptomatic cardiovascular disease, Moderate to severe hypertension, Hyperthyroidism, Known hypersensitivity or idiosyncrasy to the sympathomimetic amines, Allergy to amphetamines or to components of Vyvanse® or its container, Glaucoma, Agitated states, Patients with a history of drug abuse, During or within 14 days following the administration of monoamine oxidase inhibitors (hypertensive crises may result).

Vyvanse® should not be used in patients with symptomatic cardiovascular disease including coronary artery disease and should generally not be used in patients with known serious structural cardiac abnormalities or other serious heart problems (e.g., cardiomyopathy, serious heart rhythm abnormalities) that may place them at increased vulnerability to the sympathomimetic effects of ADHD drugs.

Please consult the Vyvanse® Product Monograph for complete prescribing information, particularly in relation to pre-existing psychosis, bipolar illness, emergence of new psychotic or manic symptoms, aggression, seizures, tics, growth suppression and visual disturbances. The misuse of amphetamines may cause serious cardiovascular adverse events and sudden death.

Adverse events reported at a frequency ≥1 %:

In the child clinical trials (patients 6–12 years old): Abdominal pain upper, vomiting, nausea, dry mouth, pyrexia, weight decreased, decreased appetite, anorexia, headache, dizziness, somnolence, psychomotor hyperactivity, insomnia, irritability, initial insomnia, affect lability, tic, obsessive-compulsive symptoms, agitation, aggression, rash, fatigue.

In the adolescent clinical trials (patients 13–17 years old): Palpitations, dry mouth, nausea, fatigue, weight decreased, blood pressure increased, decreased appetite, anorexia, headache, dizziness, tremor, insomnia, irritability, initial insomnia, affect lability, dyspnea, diarrhea, vomiting.

In the adult clinical trials (patients 18 years old and over): Palpitations, tachycardia, dry mouth, nausea, diarrhea, abdominal pain upper, feeling jittery, weight decreased, blood pressure increased, decreased appetite, anorexia, headache, tremor, insomnia, anxiety, initial insomnia, middle insomnia, agitation, restlessness, libido decreased, logorrhea, erectile dysfunction, dyspnea, hyperhidrosis, rash, dizziness, fatigue, irritability.

References

VYVANSE® Product Monograph. Shire Canada Inc.

Stanczak A and Ferra A. Prodrugs and Soft Drugs. Pharmacological Reports 2006; (58)599-613.

Pennick M. Absorption of lisdexamfetamine dimesylate and its enzymatic conversion to D-amphetamine. Neuropsychiatric Disease and Treatment 2010;6:317–27.

Pliszka SR. Comparing the effects of stimulant and non-stimulant agents on catecholamine function: implications for theories in ADHD. In: Solanto MV, Arnsten AFT, Castellanos FX, eds. Stimulant drugs and ADHD: Basic and clinical neuroscience. New York, NY: Oxford University Press; 2001:332–52.

10.5 Non-stimulant Medication

Atomoxetine (Strattera*) 10, 18, 25, 40, 60, 80, 100 mg capsules Use with ADHD patients who do not respond to, or are intolerant of, stimulant medication, or for those patients for who stimulant medication is contraindicated. **Consider as the first line if there is comorbid substance abuse, severe tic disorder or anxiety disorder**	Start with .5 mg/kg/day for children and adolescents, and 18 mg/day for adults Increase gradually to reach a maintenance dose of 1.2 mg/kg/day in children and adolescents and 60–80 mg in adults **Maximum** dose 60 mg/day for children and adolescents, and 100 mg for adults

*trade name in Canada

10.5.1 Additional Information About Medications - Nonstimulants

Atomoxetine HCl - ATX Strattera® (ATX)

Atomoxetine, a highly selective norepinephrine reuptake inhibitor, is approved for the treatment of ADHD in children, adolescents, and adults. Unlike the stimulants, ATX is not a controlled substance; therefore, clinicians can provide samples and prescribe refills. ATX acts by blocking the norepinephrine reuptake pump on the presynaptic membrane, thus increasing the availability of intrasynaptic norepinephrine. FDA approved its use for ADHD patients over the age of 6 years. Atomoxetine is especially useful for ADHD patients who do not response or develop unacceptable side effects to stimulant use. It is also helpful in ADHD patients with comorbid tics, anxiety and SUD. Atomoxetine has been shown to be effective in treating the core ADHD symptoms in children, adolescents and adults (Michelson 2001, 2002, 2003). Several reported studies have shown improved functioning, better quality of life measures, and good long-term safety after 2 years of continuous Atomoxetine use (Adler 2005, 2006; Wilens 2006; Kratochvil 2006). Atomoxetine has also been shown to be an effective treatment for ADHD patients with comorbid anxiety and depression, and it may be a reasonable initial choice for those patients (Kratochvil 2005).

Atomoxetine is usually prescribed once daily, although twice daily dosing can also be used. Atomoxetine should be initiated at doses of about 0.5 mg/kg body weight for about 2 weeks, and then titrated upward based on clinical response to 1.2 and 1.4 mg/kg, or a maximum total dose of approximately 100 mg/day. Higher doses have been used. It comes in seven doses (10, 18, 25, 40, 60, 80 and 100 mg). The capsules should never be opened as it may cause irritation of the gastric lining (Michelson 2001). It may take several weeks before the benefits from Atomoxetine become apparent; therefore, it is important to inform patients about this to ensure continued compliance despite apparent little impact on symptoms during the initial stages of treatment. Measurements of blood levels are not required. Atomoxetine undergoes extensive biotransformation, which is affected by poor metabolism by cytochrome P450 (CYP) 2D6 in a small percentage of the population; these patients have greater exposure to, and slower elimination of, Atomoxetine than extensive metabolizers. Patients with hepatic insufficiency show an increase in Atomoxetine exposure.

Common adverse effects with Atomoxetine use include gastrointestinal upset, headaches, fatigue, and mild increase in heart rate and blood pressure. Rare, but important, adverse effects that should be discussed with patients include liver toxicity and increase suicidal thoughts. Two cases of liver toxicity were reported by the manufacturer, and in both these patients with liver damage, it was completely reversible after stopping the Atomoxetine (Prince 2006). ATX should be discontinued in patients who have jaundice and patients should contact their doctors if they develop pruritus, jaundice, dark urine, right upper quadrant tenderness, or unexplained flulike symptoms. At this time, laboratory monitoring outside of routine medical care usually is not necessary (Wernicke 2002). An analysis of clinical trials by the manufacturer showed increased suicidal thoughts in 4 (0.4 %) out of 1,000 patients, but there were no attempted or completed suicides (Product Monograph). Nevertheless, the FDA warns clinicians to counsel patients about this potential risk.

10.5.2 Additional Information About Medications (Alphabetical Order) – Other Medications

Bupropion HCl – Wellbutrin® SR Wellbutrin® XL

Bupropion hydrochloride is used as an antidepressant and in smoking cessation. It blocks the reuptake of noradrenaline and dopamine (Horst 1998). It is not a controlled substance. Although it has been shown to be efficacious in the treatment of ADHD symptoms in children and adults, it is not currently approved for use in ADHD (Wilens 2002). Bupropion may be particularly useful in ADHD patients with comorbid SUD and depression, and/or nicotine use and does not cause sexual dysfunction or risk of abuse or diversion. Side effects include insomnia, headache, weight loss, and a slight increased risk of seizures. Wellbutrin® takes up to 4–6 weeks to show effect (Wilens 2001; Solkhah 2005; Levin 2002).

Clonidine

The main mechanism of action and therapeutic effects of Clonidine and Guanfacine for ADHD are not well understood. More research is needed, but animal studies suggest alpha-2 adrenergic agonists may strengthen working memory by improving functional connectivity in the prefrontal cortex (Wang 2007).

Clonidine has been used for the treatment of ADHD since the early 1990s. Systematic reviews of evidence from controlled clinical trials show that it is less effective than stimulants and likely less effective than Atomoxetine, tricyclic antidepressants, and Bupropion (Pliszka et al. 2006; Prince 2006). It is frequently used as an adjunct to stimulants to manage aggressive behavior or tics, or to improve sleep.

Common side effects include drowsiness, dry mouth, gastrointestinal upsets, hypotension and dizziness. In children and adolescents with ADHD and comorbid ODD or Conduct Disorder, methylphenidate plus Clonidine could be considered to treat the ADHD symptoms. In children and adolescents with ADHD and a comorbid tic disorder/Tourette syndrome, Clonidine should be considered if ADHD symptoms show poor response to stimulants or Atomoxetine. Discontinuation should be gradual to avoid rebound hypertension.

Guanfacine

Guanfacine is an alpha-2 adrenoreceptor agonist and is more selective for the alpha-2 receptor compared to Clonidine. This selectivity imparts less sedation and less dizziness compared with Clonidine. In a clinical trial, onset of therapeutic effect occurred between weeks 2 and 4. The most commonly reported treatment emergent adverse events were dry mouth, headache, dizziness, gastrointestinal effects, constipation, abdominal pain, dry skin and fatigue and sedation. Small to modest changes in blood pressure, heart rate and ECG parameters were observed, but were not clinically meaningful (Biederman 2008). It has been used in the treatment of ADHD, and is available in the United States.

Studies suggest that Guanfacine in combination with psychostimulants does not produce a unique side effect pattern from that reported with monotherapy of either Guanfacine or psychostimulants alone (Spencer 2009). Guanfacine also demonstrated efficacy to reduce oppositional symptoms in children with combined ADHD and oppositional behaviors (Connor 2005).

Modafinil (Alertec®)

Modafinil is a non-controlled substance defined as a CNS stimulant. It is primarily indicated for narcolepsy, sleep apnea, and shift work sleep disorders. However, it is not approved for ADHD patients by Health Canada, nor the FDA. Modafinil at 4 mg/kg/day has been shown to improve cognitive and meta-cognitive functioning in healthy, non-sleep deprived adults (Baranski 2004), and has been shown to have efficacy in the treatment of core ADHD symptoms in children (Greenhill 2006; Swanson et al. 2006).

Common side effects are headache, dry mouth, loss of appetite and weight, nausea, diarrhea, rhinitis, decreased effectiveness of hormonal birth control pills, and anxiety. Steven Johnson syndrome has been reported. There is a need for more research on Modafinil use in ADHD.

Tricyclic Antidepressants (TCA)

Tricyclic antidepressants are older antidepressants that declined in use due to risk of death with overdose. The evidence for tricyclic antidepressants (TCAs) is largely from the early 1990s and is mainly based on Imipramine/Desipramine. The TCAs are more effective in addressing the behavioral symptoms (as measured by Conners Teachers Rating Scale) than attention/concentration deficits.

Tricyclic antidepressants should not be routinely used in treatment of ADHD, and when used, electrocardiographic monitoring should be conducted before and during treatment. Caution is warranted in patients with a personal or family history of cardiac problems.

10.5.3 General Contraindication of Psychostimulants

Mixed salts of amphetamines

- MAO inhibitors within 14 days, glaucoma, symptomatic cardiovascular disease, hyperthyroidism, moderate to severe hypertension

Dextroamphetamine and Methylphenidate

- MAO inhibitors within 14 days, glaucoma, and preexisting severe gastrointestinal narrowing

Caution with anticoagulants, anticonvulsants, and phenylbutazone and tricyclic antidepressants.

10.5.4 Drug Interactions

Markowitz and his group conducted a review that indicated that co-administration of MPH and Imipramine could possibly result in increased concentrations of Impiramine. However, it appears in all likelihood that metabolically generated Desipramine concentrations are unaffected. There is also little involvement of MPH with CYP 2D.

No clinically significant interactions occurred between Desipramine and DEX.

Psychostimulants increase the level of Phenytoin, Carbamazepine, and Phenobarbital. At the same time, these antiepileptics may lower the level psychostimulants as they act as universal enzyme inducer.

Psychostimulants increase the level of MAO inhibitor, SSRI and TCAs.

Psychostimulants may increase the effect of Warfarin.

In absence of Schizophrenia, co-administration of antipsychotic agents with psychostimulants may be expected to result in only some mutual antagonism of central dopaminergic effects.

General References and Related Reading

Adler LA, Spencer TJ, Milton DR et al (2005) Long term, open-label study of the safety and efficacy of atomoxetine in adults with attention-deficit hyperactivity disorder: an interim analysis. J Clin Psychiatry 66(3):294–299

Adler LA, Spencer TJ, Faraone SV et al (2006) Atomoxetine and adult attention-deficit/hyperactivity disorder: the effects of comorbidity. J Clin Psychiatry 67(3):415–420

Baranski JV, Pigeau R, Dinich P et al (2004) Effects of modafinil on cognitive and meta-cognitive performance. Hum Psychopharmacol 19(5):323–332

Biederman J, Balderssarini RJ, Wright V et al (1989) A double-bind placebo controlled study of Desipramine in the treatment of attention deficit disorder: I. Efficacy. J Am Acad Child Adolesc Psychiatry 28:777–784

Biederman J, Melmed RD, Patel A et al (2008) A randomized, double-blind, placebo-controlled study of Guanfacine extended release in children and adolescents with attention-deficit hyperactivity disorder. Pediatrics 121(1):e73–e84

CADDRA (2011) Canadian ADHD Practice Guidelines [online] In: Umesh J, Hechtman L et al., editors. www.caddra.ca

Childress AC, Berry SA (2012) Pharmacotherapy of attention-deficit hyperactivity disorder in adolescents. Drugs 72(3):309–325

Coghil D (2011) Pragmatic measures in paediatric psychopharmacology – are we getting it right? Eur Neuropsychopharmacol 21(8):571–583

Conners CK, Casat CD, Gualtieri CT et al (1996) Burpropion hydrochloride in attention deficit disorder with hyperactivity. J Am Acad Child Adolesc Psychiatry 35:1314–1321

Connor DF (2005) Psychostimulants in attention deficit hyperactivity disorder. In: Gozal D, Molfese DL, editors. Attention deficit hyperactivity disorder: from genes to patients. New Jersey: Humana Press, pp. 487–527

Connor DF, Findling RL, Kollins SH et al (2010) Effects of Guanfacine extended release, a non-scheduled alpha 1A-adrenoceptor agonist, on oppositional symptoms in children aged 6 to 12 years with a diagnosis of attention-deficit hyperactivity disorder and the presence of oppositional symptom. CNS Drugs 24(9):755–768

Daughton JM, Kratochvil CJ (2009) Review of ADHD pharmacotherapies: advantages, disadvantages, and clinical pearls. J Am Acad Child Adoloesc Psychiatry 48(3):240–248

Davidson MA (2008) ADHD in adults: a review of the literature. J Atten Disord 11(6):628–641

Dopheide JA, Pliszka SR (2009) Attention-deficit hyperactivity disorder: an update. Pharmacotherapy 29(6):656–679

Findling RL (2008) Evolution of the treatment of attention-deficit hyperactivity disorder in children: a review. Clin Ther 30(5):942–957

Garnock-Jones KP, Keating GM (2010) Spotlight on Atomoxetine in attention-deficit hyperactivity disorder in children and adolsecents. CNS Drugs 24(1):85–88

Graham J, Coghill D (2008) Adverse effects of pharmacotherapies for attention-deficit hyperactivity disorder: epidemiology, prevention and management. CNS Drugs 22(3):231–237

Greenhill LL, Biederman J, Boellner SW (2002) A randomized, double-blind, placebo-controlled study of Modafinil film-coated tablets in children and adolescents with attention-deficit hyperactivity disorder. J Am Acad Child Adolesc Psychiatry 45(5):503–511

Greenhill L, Kollins S et al (2006) Efficacy and safety of immediate-release methylphenidate treatment for preschoolers with ADHD. J Am Acad Child Adolesc Psychiatry 45(11):1284–93

Horst WD, Preskorn SH (1998) Mechanisms of action and clinical characteristic of three atypical antidepressants: venlafaxine, nefazodone, bupropion. J Affect Disord 51:237–254

Huang YS, Tsai MH (2001) Long-term outcomes with medications for attention-deficit hyperactivity disorder: current status of knowledge. CNS Drugs 25(7):539–554, Erratum in: CNS Drugs. 2011 Nov. 1, 25(11): 932, Dosage error in article text

Humphreys C, Carcia-Bournissen F, Ito S, Koren G (2007) Exposure to attention deficit hyperactivity disorder medications during pregnancy. Can Fam Physician 53(7):1153–1155

Kaplan G, Newcorn JH (2011) Pharmacotherapy for child and adolescent attention-deficit hyperactivity disorder. Pediatr Clin N Am 58(1):99–120, xi

Kolar D (2008) Treatment of adults with attention-deficit/hyperactivity disorder. Neuropsychiatr Dis Treat 4(2):389–403

Kratochvil DJ, Newcorn JH, Arnold LE (2005) Atomoxetine alone or combined with fluoxetine for treating ADHD with comorbid depressive or anxiety symptoms. J Am Acad Child Adolesc Psychiatry 44(9):915–924

Kratochvil CJ, Wilens TE, Grennhill LL et al (2006) Effects of long term Atomoxetine treatment for young children with attention-deficit hyperactivity disorder. J Am Acad Child Adolesc Psychiatry 45(8):919–927

Levin FR, Evans SM, McDowell DM et al (2002) Bupropion treatment for cocaine abuse and adult attention-deficit hyperactivity disorder. J Addict Disord 21(2):1–16

Lin JS, Gervansoni D, Hou Y et al (2000) Effects of amphetamine and Modafinil on the sleep/wake cycle during experimental hypersomnia induces by sleep deprivation in the cat. J Sleep Res 9(1):89–96

Meijer WM, Faber A, van den Ban E, Tobi H (2009) Current issues around the pharmacotherapy of ADHD in children and adults. Pharm World Sci 31(5):509–516, Epub 2009 Jun 27

Michelson D, Faries DE, Wernicke J et al (2001) Atomoxetine in the treatment of children and adolescents with attention-deficit hyperactivity disorder: a randomized, placebo controlled, dose–response study. Pediatrics 108(5):E83

Michelson D, Kratochvil CJ, Heligenstein JH et al (2002) Atomoxetine and methylphenidate treatment in children with ADHD: A prospective, randomized, open-label trial. J Am Acad Child Adolesc Psychiatry 41(7):776–784

Michelson D, Adler L, Spencer T et al (2003) Atomoxetine in adults with ADHD: two randomized, placebo-controlled studies. Biol Psychiatry 53(2):112–120

Murray DW (2010) Treatment of preschoolers with attention-deficit/hyperactivity disorder. Curr Psychiatry Rep 12(5):374–381

Pliszka SR et al (2006) Texas Consensus Conference Panel on Pharmacotherapy of childhood attention deficit hyperactivity disorder. The Texas Childrens' Medication Algorithm Project: revision of the algorithm for pharmacotherapy of attention-deficit hyperactivity disorder. J Am Acad Child Adolesc Psychiatry 45(6):642–657

Pliszka S (2007) AACAP Work Group on Quality Issues. Practice parameter for the assessment and treatment of children and adolescents with attention-deficit/hyperactivity disorder. J Am Acad Child Adolesc Psychiatry 46(7):894–921

Prince JB (2006) Pharmacotherapy of attention-deficit hyperactivity disorder in children and adolescents: update on new stimulant preparations, Atomoxetine, and novel treatments. Child Adolesc Psychiatr Clin N Am 15(1):13–50

Pringsheim T, Steeves T (2011) Pharmacological treatment for attention deficit hyperactivity disorder (ADHD) in children with comorbid tic disorders. Cochrane Database Syst Rev (4): CD007900

Rostain AL (2008) Attention-deficit hyperactivity disorder in adults: evidence-based recommendations for management. Postgrad Med 120(3):27–38

Safety and side effect information in children, teens and adults (2011). http://www.strattera.com

Salle FR, McGough J, Wigel T et al (2009) Guanfacine extended release in children and adolescents with attention-deficit hyperactivity disorder: a placbo-controlled trial. J Am Acad Child Adolesc Psychiatry 48(2):155–165

Sallee FR, Eaton K (2010) Guanfacine extended-release for attention-deficit hyperactivity disorder (ADHD). Expert Opin Pharmacother 11(15):2549–2556

Santosh PJ, Sattar S, Canagaratnam M (2011) Efficacy and tolerability of pharmacotherapies for attention-deficit hyperactivity disorder in adults. CNS Drugs 25(9):737–763

Schachar R, Ickowicz A, Crosbie J et al (2008) Cognitive and behavioral effects of multilayer-release methylphenidate in the treatment of children with attention-deficit hyperactivity disorder. J Child Adolesc Psychopharmacol 18(1):11–24
Slatkoff J, Greenfiled B (2006) Pharmacological treatment of attention-deficit hyperactivity disorder in adults. Expert Opin Investig Drugs 15(6):649–667
Solkhah R, Wilens TE, Daly J et al (2005) Burpropion SR for the treatment of substance-abusing outpatient adolescents with attention-deficit hyperactivity disorder and mood disorders. J Child Adolesc Psychopharmacol 15(5):777–786
Spencer TJ, Greenbaum M, Ginsger LD, Murphy WR (2009) Safety and effectiveness of co-administration of Guanfacine extended release and psychostimulants in children and adolescents with attention-deficit hyperactivity disorder. J Child Adolesc Psychopharmacol 19(5):501–510
Swanson JM, Greenhill LL, Lopez FA et al (2006) Modafinil film-coated tablets in children and adolescents with attention – deficit hyperactivity disorder: results of a randomized, double-blind, placebo-controlled fixed-dose study followed by abrupt discontinuation. J Clin Psychiatry 67(1):137–147
Turner DC, Clark L, Dowson J et al (2004) Modafinil improves cognition and response inhibition in adult attention-deficit hyperactivity disorder. Biol Psychiatry 55(10):1031–1040
Vitiello B (2008) Understanding the risk of using medications for attention deficit hyperactivity disorder with respect to physical growth and cardiovascular function. Child Adolesc Psychiatr Clin N Am 17(2):459–474, xi
Wang Y, Zheng Y, Du Y et al (2007) Atomoxetine versus methylphenidate in paediatric outpatients with attention deficit hyperactivity disorder: a randomized, double-blind comparison trial. Aust N Z J Psychiatry 41(3):222–30
Wernicke JF, Kratochvil CJ (2002) Safety profile of Atomoxetine in the treatment of children and adolescents with ADHD. J Clin Psychiatry 63(12):50–55
Wigal SB (2009) Efficacy and safety limitations of attention-deficit hyperactivity disorder pharmacotherapy in children and adults. CNS Drugs 23(1):21–31
Wigal SB, Cahe S, Patel A, Steinberg-Epstein R (2010) Advances in the treatment of attention-deficit hyperactivity disorder: a guide for pediatric neurologists. Semin Pediatr Neurol 17(4):230–236
Wilens TE (2006) Mechanism of action of agents used in attention-deficit hyperactivity disorder. J Clin Psychiatry 67(8):32–38
Wilens TE, Spencer TJ (2010) Understanding attention-deficit/hyperactivity disorder from childhood to adulthood. Postgrad Med 122(5):97–109
Wilens TE, Spencer TJ, Biederman J et al (2001) A controlled clinical trial of bupropion for attention deficit hyperactivity disorder in adults. Am J Psychiatry 158(2):282–288
Wilens TE, Spencer TJ, Biederman J (2002) Attention deficit/hyperactivity disorder across the life span. Ann Rev Med 53:113–131
Wilens TE, Newcorn JJ, Kratochovil CJ et al (2006) Long term Atomoxetine treatment in adolescents with attention-deficit hyperactivity disorder. J Pediatr 146(1):112–119
Wolraich ML et al (2005) Attention-deficit hyperactivity disorder among adolescents: a review of the diagnosis, treatment and clinical implications. Pediatrics 115(6):1734–1746

ADHD Guidelines Available on the Internet

American Psychological Association. http://www.apa.org/topics/adhd/index.aspx
Australian ADHD Draft Guidelines. http://www.nhmrc.gov.au/guidelines/publications/ch54
Canadian ADHD Guidelines. http://www.caddra.ca/cms4/
National Institute for Health and Clinical Excellence (NICE). http://publications.nice.org.uk/attention-deficit-hyperactivity-disorder-cg72
Scottish ADHD Guidelines. http://www.sign.ac.uk/guidelines/fulltext/112/index.html

11 Management of Adverse Events

Adverse effects of stimulant medications include decreased appetite, sleep disturbance, headaches, irritability, nervousness, stomach upset, abdominal pain, nausea, abdominal discomfort, weight loss, tearfulness, stuttering, dizziness, increased heart rate and blood pressure.

More severe side effects (rare) can include psychotic symptoms and sensitivity reactions that will require discontinuation of the medication.

Special consideration had been given to the impact of ADHD medications on growth, tics, seizure, cardiac events and primary active psychotic disorders.

11.1 Contraindications of Psychostimulants

Stimulants are generally contraindicated in individuals with untreated thyroid dysfunction particularly hyperthyroidism, pheochromocytoma, glaucoma, known hypersensitivity or idiosyncrasy to the sympathetic amines and concurrent treatment (or treatment within 14 days) with monoamine oxidase inhibitors (MAO) and active substance use. Stimulants are also contraindicated in patients with significant heart disease hypertension and potential to increase the risk of sudden cardiac death (e.g., coronary artery disease, structural heart disease, cardiomyopathy, history of arrhythmia and untreated hypertension).

11.2 Management of Side Effects

- **Cardiovascular risk**
  - In May 2006, Health Canada issued important safety information on ADHD medications and recommended that ADHD drugs should be started at the lowest possible dose, and increased slowly, as individual patient response to these drugs is known to vary widely. The recommendation also stated that:

J. Sadek, *A Clinician's Guide to ADHD*,

DOI 10.1007/978-3-319-02359-5_11,

  - ADHD drugs should not be used if a patient has:
    - Symptomatic cardiac disease;
    - Moderate to severe hypertension;
    - Advance arteriosclerosis, coronary artery disease; or
    - Hyperthyroidism
- Generally, ADHD drugs should not be used in patients with known structural cardiac abnormalities. Before prescribing an ADHD drug, it is important to be aware of whether the patient has:
  - a family history of sudden death, or death related to cardiac problems;
  - participates in strenuous exercise; or
  - takes other sympathomimetic drugs

  These are thought to be additional risk factors. In patients with relevant risk factors, and based on the physician's judgment, further evaluation of the cardiovascular system may be considered before starting on the drug.
- American Heart Association recommends that before beginning therapy of stimulant medications, careful history should be obtained with special attention to symptoms, such as palpitations, syncope, or near syncope. Medications use, such as other prescribed and over-the-counter medications, should be determined. The family history should be reviewed with reference to the long QT Syndrome or other causes of sudden, unexplained death. Detection of these symptoms, or risk factors, warrants a cardiovascular evaluation by a pediatric cardiologist before initiation of therapy.
- Patients who are considered to need long-term treatment with ADHD drugs should undergo periodic evaluation of their cardiovascular status, based on the physician's judgment.
- Patients taking drugs for the management of ADHD should be advised not to discontinue their medications without consultation with their physician.
- At follow-up visits, patients receiving psychotropic drug therapy should be questioned about the addition of any drugs, and the occurrence of any of the above symptoms. The physical examination should include determination of heart rate and blood pressure.
- ECG is not routinely recommended before starting stimulant medications.
- Risk of sudden death is found to be similar to the general population.

- **Growth and appetite suppression**
  - Treatment with psychostimulant medications may result in a reduction in both height and weight. On average, the reduction in height amounts to approximately 1 cm per year during the first 1–3 years of treatment and 3 kg less than predicted over a year period.
  - In the majority of cases, these effects are usually minor and the majority of patients fall within the 95 % of the population. The small group that suffer from significant growth suppression usually show a dose dependent effect with doses over 1.5 mg per kilogram per day (given continuously) resulting in more problems; preschool children may be particularly vulnerable to growth effects.
  - Reduced caloric intake and suboptimal nutrition due to appetite suppression are the more likely causes of most growth suppression. Other hypotheses considered were the dysregulation of receptors in the growth system, effect of

ADHD on growth hormone, prolactin and possible increase or decrease in growth related to ADHD itself.

- Monitor growth (weight and height) closely and use the growth charts.
- Simple strategies that might be helpful:
  - Consuming additional meals, or snacks, early in the morning or late in the evening when the stimulant effects of the drug have worn off;
  - Obtaining dietary advice *(please see the end of this chapter, after references, for nutrition information from the Scottish Guidelines)*;
  - Consuming high calorie foods of good nutritional value;
  - Changing the timing of the dose and/or meals;
  - Consuming high energy snacks;
  - If growth is significantly affected by drug treatment (that is, the child or young person has not met the height expected for their age), the option of a planned break in treatment over school holidays may be considered to allow "catch-up" growth to occur. Drug holidays can be planned. Current data does not support specific guidelines indicating what magnitude of height or weight gain deceleration should trigger changes in the treatment regimen.
  - If there is evidence of weight loss associated with drug treatment in adults with ADHD, clinicians should consider monitoring body mass index and changing the drug if weight loss persists.
  - In children, you can follow the medical criteria for referral to pediatric endocrinologist to consider growth hormone therapy in treatment of short stature, particularly if the height is more than two standard deviations below the population mean for the age, and a 1 year decrease of more than .5 standard deviation in height. Consideration should also be given to the mother and father's height.

- **Jaundice, signs of liver disease or biliary obstruction**
  - Stop medication immediately and seek the help of a specialist.
- **Psychotic symptoms**
  - New onset psychotic symptoms that develop during the course of treatment of ADHD should be carefully evaluated. Development of psychosis as a side effect of psychostimulant is very rare, and in most cases, the impact of psychotic adverse events is mild and mostly self-limiting. As indicated in the Australian and UK guidelines, caution would be appropriate when prescribing ADHD drugs to children and young people with a family history of psychosis, or past history of psychotic episodes. A full psychiatric assessment should be conducted to determine if the psychotic symptoms are primary or secondary. A determination of starting an antipsychotic should be made at that point.
- **Seizures**
  - Despite the thin evidence of ADHD treatment in children with seizure disorder, it is not a contraindication to treat ADHD in the presence of seizure disorder.
  - New onset seizure has been observed after starting a few patients on ADHD medications, and ADHD patients have been shown to have incidence rates of unprovoked seizures and epilepsy two or three times greater than non-ADHD

children. After careful evaluation, some patients who had documented seizure may start an antiepileptic medication.
  - If seizures are exacerbated in a child or young person with epilepsy, or de novo seizures emerge following introduction of stimulant or Atomoxetine, another approach is to discontinue the drug and trial a different class.
  - It is important to rule out the possibility of substance abuse inducing seizure in patients with ADHD.
  - Some studies support the lowering of seizure threshold with the use of psychostimulants but other studies found no evidence for an increase in relative risk for either MPH (.8) or Atomoxetine (1.1)
  - Fatal hepatotoxicity has been reported as an extremely rare event in young epileptic children with polypharmacy or inborn errors of metabolism, and the combination of Atomoxetine with antiepileptic agents that might increase the risk of liver toxicity. Requires close clinical monitoring.
  - ADHD symptoms in epilepsy may be improved by non-specific interventions, such as better seizure control, decreasing AED polypharmacy, reducing drug interactions, and switching to AEDs with fewer cognitive and behavioral effects epilepsy.
- **Sleep disturbance**
  - Some clinicians concluded from several studies that the effect of ADHD medication on sleep may be beneficial, at least in some patients, but further research with more subjects, and with a variety of medication, is needed. Many patients treated with psychostimulants complain of insomnia, so an approach to manage this problem is necessary. Clinicians should document sleep patterns and complaints before treatment to help interpret problems that may arise after medication has been prescribed.
  - Sleep hygiene, consisting of simple behavioral approaches that promote sound sleep (e.g., creating a restful environment and avoiding caffeine), is a primary approach for most patients with insomnia.
  - It might be helpful to look into shifting the dose to an earlier time or reducing an existing evening dose.
  - Mirtazapine 15 mg HS has been reported as safe and effective for adults taking psychostimulants.
  - Atomoxetine may have an effect on sleep that is different from that of psychostimulants, including reduced sleep latency, but less efficiency. In a randomized, double-blinded, crossover trial, Methylphenidate treatment for children with ADHD caused more initial insomnia, but fewer awakenings compared with Atomoxetine treatment. Switching to Atomoxetine may be considered for patients who prefer it, or who do not respond to adjunctive interventions for stimulant-associated insomnia.
  - Melatonin 3–6 mg at least half hour before sleep can be used. Other pharmacological options include: Zopiclone 7.5 mg HS, Trazodone 25–50 mg HS, Benzodiazepines, such as Lorazepam, (consider, though, the high addiction potential), Methotrimeprazine 10–15 mg HS, or Quetiapine 25 mg HS for some resistant cases.

- **Suicide**
  - First, assess the suicide as a separate issue. Determine whether the patient is expressing suicidal ideation, intent, plan or is there a history of chronic self-harm behavior as in a personality disorder. Evaluate if suicide developed after starting Atomoxetine (more risk) or psychostimulant medications. Suicide prevention should be the first priority over any other consideration. You can use a tool, such as the Nova Scotia Suicide Risk Assessment Tool, to determine the risk level and management strategy. It is important to document all your findings about suicide and communicate them to others involved in the care of the patient. Caution is required when prescribing ADHD drugs to children and young adults with a past history of serious suicide attempts or depression. Families and caregivers should be advised of the need to recognize any emergence of emotional change, or self-injurious thinking, and to communicate well with the prescriber.
  - Patients being treated with ADHD drugs should be observed for the emergence of suicide-related events. If they do emerge in treatment, consideration should be given to dose reduction and/or other changes in therapeutic regimen, including the possibility of discontinuing medication, especially if symptoms are severe or abrupt in onset, or were not part of the patient's presenting symptoms.
- **Tics**
  - Tic Disorder is not a contraindication for psychostimulant use; however, several patients may suffer from worsening of tics. Taking a history, and closely monitoring comorbid tics is needed. It is important to note that several literature reviews suggested that stimulants are adequately safe in patients with both ADHD and Tic Disorder since tics are naturally waxing and waning. It is often difficult to decide if worsening of tics is provoked by the ADHD medication.
  - Treatment of both Tics and ADHD symptoms can be treated together by adding antipsychotic medication to the psychostimulant or Atomoxetine. The alpha-2 adrenergic agonist Clonidine and Guanfacine have been showing promise in the treatment of tics, particularly in combination with stimulant medications.

For information on Alternative Therapies that have been researched or tested, please see the end of this chapter, after references, for excerpt of information from the Scottish Guidelines.

11.3 Common Side Effects and Contraindications - Atomoxetine

- The common adverse effects associated with ATX include decreased appetite, drowsiness, abdominal pain, nausea and vomiting, dizziness, increased heart rate and blood pressure.
- Less common side effects include dyspepsia and mood swings. There have been three published case reports of severe liver injury in children and adults using ATX. These individuals recovered when the drug was discontinued.

Suicide-related behavior (suicide attempts and suicidal ideation) has been reported in patients treated with Atomoxetine.

- Atomoxetine is contraindicated for people with narrow-angle glaucoma and concurrent treatment (or treatment within 14 days) with monoamine oxidase inhibitors (MAO). It is also contraindicated in people with structural cardiac abnormalities, symptomatic cardiovascular disease, or other serious heart problems as it increases the heart rate and the blood pressure.

Alternative Approaches from Scottish Guidelines

The following is directly from the Scottish Guidelines; please refer to the permission listing at the beginning of the book.

Nutrition and Complementary and alternative Therapies

<u>Nutrition</u>

This section examines the evidence base for dietary manipulation and supplementation as an alternative or complementary intervention in the treatment of core ADHD/HKD symptoms. Investigation of the role of dietary factors in the causation of ADHD/HKD was outside the guideline remit.

8.1.1 food additives

There is evidence from well controlled studies that some food colourants and preservatives can have adverse behavioural effects on children both in the general population and in those diagnosed with ADHD/HKD.[134,135]

In two studies in non-clinical populations of children aged three years and eight/nine years, mixed artificial colourants (sunset yellow, tartrazine, carmoisine and ponceau 4R) or the preservative sodium benzoate, or both, exacerbated hyperactive behaviours as rated by parents.

The nature of the response is individual and appears to have a pharmacological rather than an allergic mechanism.[136,137]

A meta-analysis of additive-free diets followed by food challenges in children with hyperactive disorders showed that pathological responses to foods were multiple and idiosyncratic although the most common responses were to the artificial colourant tartrazine and the preservative sodium benzoate.[138]

Avoiding foods and drinks that contain certain artificial colours and/or preservatives may help some children with ADHD/HKD. Parents should be advised to take reasonable steps to limit the number and variety of these in their children's diets, excluding any item that seems to provoke an extreme physical or behavioural reaction.

8.1.2 omega-3 and omega-6 fatty acid supplementation

Three systematic reviews of studies of the effectiveness of fatty acid supplementation in children with ADHD/HKD reported a range of methodological difficulties in the trials included.[134,138,139]

No consistent evidence was identified and meta-analysis of study results was not possible.

8.1.3 iron supplementation

In a small ($n = 23$) well conducted, placebo controlled RCT of ferrous sulphate supplementation in French school children with ADHD/HKD who had low ferritin stores but were not clinically anaemic, there were significant decreases in symptom scores over 12 weeks (ADHD/HKD Rating Scale, $p < 0.008$; Clinical Global Impression Scale, $p < 0.01$).[140]

Clinicians should consider iron status when taking a history, with measurement of serum iron and ferritin, and treatment, where appropriate.

8.1.4 zinc supplementation

A single RCT on zinc sulphate monotherapy as a treatment for ADHD/HKD found a significant therapeutic response but the validity of these findings was compromised by a high drop-out rate.[141]

A small study ($n = 44$) examining the effect of zinc supplementation on the response to methylphenidate in medication-naive children with ADHD/HKD, found that the group taking methylphenidate and zinc improved significantly more than those on methylphenidate and placebo as judged by Du Paul scale parent ratings ($p < 0.048$) and teacher ratings ($p = 0.04$).[142]

There is insufficient evidence on which to base a recommendation.

8.1.5 antioxidants

One controlled study was identified using the antioxidant Pycnogenol®, derived from maritime pine bark, in children diagnosed with a hyperkinetic disorder or attention deficit disorder. A significant effect on hyperactivity scores compared with the baseline and a placebo was seen after one month on treatment. The effects disappeared after a further month without treatment.[143]

This trial has not been replicated.

8.2 complementary and alternative therapies

There is insufficient evidence on which to base any recommendations for complementary or alternative therapies in the treatment of ADHD.

8.2.1 bach flower remedies

One small placebo controlled RCT found no effect for Bach flower remedies (five flower essences) in the treatment of children with ADHD/HKD.[144]

8.2.2 homeopathy

A well conducted Cochrane meta-analysis identified four small trials of homeopathic treatments.

The study concluded that there is little evidence of efficacy.[145]

8.2.3 massage therapy

One small, short term RCT study found that twice weekly massage therapy improved short term mood state and classroom behaviour in young people with ADHD/HKD.[146]

8.2.4 neurofeedback

Neurofeedback is presently considered to be an experimental intervention in children and young people with ADHD/HKD. There are no standardised interventions.[147,148]

Related references from Scottish Guidelines

134. Rojas NL, Chan E. Old and new controversies in the alternative treatment of attention-deficit hyperactivity disorder. Mental Retardation & Developmental Disabilities Research Reviews 2005;11(2):116–30.

135. Schab DW, Trinh NH. Do artificial food colors promote hyperactivity in children with hyperactive syndromes? A metaanalysis of double-blind placebo-controlled trials. Journal of Developmental & Behavioral Pediatrics 2004;25(6):423–34.

136. Bateman B, Warner JO, Hutchinson E, Dean T, Rowlandson P, Grant C, et al. The effects of a double blind, placebo controlled, artificial food colourings and benzoate preservative challenge on hyperactivity in a general population sample of preschool children. Archives of Disease in Childhood 2004;89(6):506–11.

137. McCann D, Barrett A, Cooper A, Crumpler D, Dalen L, Grimshaw K, et al. Food additives and hyperactive behaviour in 3-year-old and 8/9-year-old children in the community: a randomised, double-blinded, placebo-controlled trial. Lancet 2007;370(9598):1560–7.

138. Benton D. The impact of diet on anti-social, violent and criminal behaviour. Neuroscience and Biobehavioral Reviews 2007;31(5):752–74.

139. Clayton EH, Hanstock TL, Garg ML, Hazell PL. Long chain omega-3 polyunsaturated fatty acids in the treatment of psychiatric illnesses in children and adolescents. Acta Neuropsychiatrica 2007;19(2):92–103.

140. Konofal E, Lecendreux M, Deron J, Marchand M, Cortese S, Zaim M, et al. Effects of iron supplementation on attention deficit hyperactivity disorder in children. Pediatr Neurol 2008;38(1):20–6.

141. Bilici M, Yildirim F, Kandil S, Bekarolu M, Yildirmi S, Deer O, et al. Double-blind, placebo-controlled study of zinc sulfate in the treatment of attention deficit hyperactivity disorder. Progress in Neuro-Psychopharmacology and Biological Psychiatry 2004;28(1):181–90.

142. Akhondzadeh S MM, Khademi M. Zinc sulphate as an adjunct to methylphenidate for the treatment of attentiondeficit hyperactivity disorder in children: a double blind and randomised trail. BMC Psychiatry 2004;4:9.

143. Trebaticka J, Kopasova S, Hradecna Z, Cinovsky K, Skodacek I, Suba J, et al. Treatment of ADHD with French maritime pine bark extract, Pycnogenol. Eur Child Adolesc Psychiatry 2006;15(6):329–35.

144. Pintov S, Hochman M, Livne A, Heyman E, Lahat E. Bach flower remedies used for attention deficit hyperactivity disorder in children - a prospective double blind controlled study. European Journal of Paediatric Neurology 2005;9(6):395–8.

145. Coulter MK, Dean ME. Homeopathy for attention deficit/hyperactivity disorder or hyperkinetic disorder. Cochrane Database of Systematic Reviews. 2007(4):(CD005648).

146. Khilnani S, Field T, Hernandez-Reif M, Schanberg S. Massage therapy improves mood and behavior of students with attentiondeficit/hyperactivity disorder. Adolescence 2003;38(152):623

147. Beauregard M, Levesque J. Functional magnetic resonance imaging investigation of the effects of neurofeedback training on the neural bases of selective attention and response inhibition in children with attention-deficit/hyperactivity disorder. Ap1plied Psychophysiology & Biofeedback 2006;31(1):3–20.

148. Baydala L, Wikman E. The efficacy of neurofeedback in the management of children with attention deficit/hyperactivity disorder. Paediatrics and Child Health 2001;6(7):451–5.

General References and Recommended Readings

Australian draft guidelines 2009

Brown RT, Amler RW, Freeman WS, Perrin JM, Stein MT, Feldman HM, Pierce K, Wolraich ML, American Academy of Pediatrics Committee on Quality Improvement; American Academy of Pediatrics Subcommittee on Attention-Deficit/Hyperactivity Disorder (2005) Treatment of attention-deficit/hyperactivity disorder: overview of the evidence. Pediatrics 115(6):e749–e757

Gibson AP, Bettinger TL, Patel NC, Crismon ML (2006) Atomoxetine versus stimulants for treatment of attention deficit/hyperactivity disorder. Ann Pharmacother 40(6):1134–1142

Harpin VA (2008) Medication options when treating children and adolescents with ADHD: interpreting the NICE guidance 2006. Arch Dis Child Educ Pract Ed 93(2):58–65

Jensen P (2002) Longer term effects of stimulant treatments for attention-deficit/hyperactivity disorder. J Atten Disord 6(1):45–56

Klein-Schwartz W (2002) Abuse and toxicity of methylphenidate. Curr Opin Pediatr 14(2):219–223

Kollins SH (2008) A qualitative review of issues arising in the use of psycho-stimulant medications in patients with ADHD and co-morbid substance use disorders. Curr Med Res Opin 24(5):1345–1357. Epub 2008 Apr 1

Kratochvil CJ, Lake M, Pliszka SR, Walkup JT (2005) Pharmacological management of treatment-induced insomnia in ADHD. J Am Acad Child Adolesc Psychiatry 44(5):499–501

NICE guidelines

Pringsheim T, Steeves T (2011) Pharmacological treatment for attention deficit hyperactivity disorder (ADHD) in children with comorbid tic disorders. Cochrane Database Syst Rev (4):CD007990

Reeves G, Schweitzer J (2004) Pharmacological management of attention-deficit hyperactivity disorder. Expert Opin Pharmacother 5(6):1313–1320

Schonwald A, Lechner E (2006) Attention deficit/hyperactivity disorder: complexities and controversies. Curr Opin Pediatr 18(2):189–195

Stiefel G, Besag FM (2010) Cardiovascular effects of methylphenidate, amphetamines and atomoxetine in the treatment of attention-deficit hyperactivity disorder. Drug Saf 33(10):821–842

www.caddra.ca

ADHD Guidelines Available on the Internet

American Psychological Association: http://www.apa.org/topics/adhd/index.aspx

Australian ADHD Draft Guidelines: http://www.nhmrc.gov.au/guidelines/publications/ch54

Canadian ADHD Guidelines: http://www.caddra.ca/cms4/

National Institute for Health and Clinical Excellence (NICE): http://publications.nice.org.uk/attention-deficit-hyperactivity-disorder-cg72

Scottish ADHD Guidelines: http://www.sign.ac.uk/guidelines/fulltext/112/index.html

Psychosocial Treatment of ADHD

12

12.1 Introduction

Management of ADHD is viewed as a multimodal approach that involves medications, medical management, educational and vocational, and behavioral interventions. Some authors suggest that the clinical benefits of medications are not extended to all areas of impairment or patients may be unresponsive or intolerant of medications, others suggest that most presentations of ADHD in children and adults are associated with behavioral problems and comorbid psychiatric disorders. Therefore, a complete and comprehensive therapeutic intervention devised for a given individual should include non-pharmacological therapies that are evidence based.

Today there is a strong agreement in the literature that psychosocial treatment is an integral component of ADHD management across a life span. Combination of medication and psychosocial treatments are being used in many treatment settings.

12.2 Overview – Children

Specifically for children, a complete and thorough assessment of the strengths and weaknesses of the child, and his/her environment (e.g., family, peer group, classroom setting) is needed so that treatments can target the specific needs of the child, their parents and other environmental contributors to the problem behavior across multiple settings (CADDRA). A psychosocial treatment plan can be family based, school based, academic based and peer based.

***Australian Draft Guidelines Recommendations – Psychosocial Interventions:* (Please refer to the copyright permission given at the beginning of the book.)**

Preschool-Aged Children (3–5 Years)

- *Structured parenting programs with demonstrated effectiveness could be considered for preschoolers with ADHD and associated behavioral problems.*
- *In considering the use of psychosocial interventions, availability, the family's resources and their capacity to adhere to the program should be taken into account.*

J. Sadek, *A Clinician's Guide to ADHD*,
DOI 10.1007/978-3-319-02359-5_12, © Springer International Publishing Switzerland 2014

School-Aged Children and Adolescents

- *Structured parenting programs with demonstrated effectiveness could be considered for children with ADHD and associated behavioral problems.*
- *Used alone, clinic-based social stalls training is not recommended for improving social skills in children with ADHD (weak evidence).*
- *There are insufficient research data to recommend the use of cognitive behavioral therapy (CBT) or family therapy for the treatment of ADHD (weak evidence).*
- *Cognitive behavioral therapy (CBT) or family therapy, may, however, be useful in addressing certain comorbidities, including anxiety, ODD and CD.*
- *For older adolescents with functional impairments associated with ADHD, the cognitive behavioral therapy (CBT) strategies described for adults may prove beneficial.*

Please also see NICE Guidelines in detail at: http://guidance.nice.org.uk/CG72/Guidance

And shorter version at: http://guidance.nice.org.uk/CG72/NICEGuidance/pdf/English

12.3 Psychosocial Interventions – Children

- **Psychoeducation**

  Psychoeducation regarding the nature, causes, diagnostic criteria, treatment, and natural history of ADHD is important in aiding parents and caregivers to cope with the behavioral and emotional sequelae associated with ADHD, to understand and implement management plans, and to anticipate difficulties.

  Parent psychoeducation is more effective if the therapist devotes more than one session to education, and more effective if the therapist educates parents about ADHD across multiple settings (e.g. home school, playground, etc.). Other areas of psychoeducation can also include strategy instruction, self-talk and organizational skill development. Topics might also include information on sleep management, anger management, and organizational skills. Handouts should be provided on ADHD identification and management, and should include resources for websites, books, local community resources, support groups and parent training for ADHD.
- **Family based intervention (Behavioral Parent Training)**

  According to the review by Chronis (2004) and Daly (2007), behavioral parent training has a long, successful history as part of a multimodal treatment approach for children with ADHD.

  ADHD may influence the functioning of the parent-child relationship, as well as increase stress in caregivers of children with the disorder leading to maladaptive coping (Wells et al. 2006). Behavioral parent training interventions are based on teaching the child more socially acceptable behavior by training primary caregivers in contingency management strategies, emphasizing behavior modifications, cues, and consequences, reward systems, and discipline (Chronis et al. 2004).

  Parents learn how to identify and manipulate the antecedents and consequences of a child's behavior; target and monitor problematic behaviors; reward acceptable social behavior through praise, positive attention, and tangible rewards; and decrease unwanted behavior through planned ignoring, time out and other non-physical discipline techniques (Chronis et al. 2006; Daly et al. 2007).

Behavioral parent training also has been found to increase parental knowledge of ADHD and caregivers' sense of competence in responding to their children, reduce parental and family stress and improve maladaptive parenting behavior (Chronis et al. 2004). It has also been associated with positive outcomes in child behavior problems, parenting skills and competence and parental conflict (Daly et al. 2007).

Several studies confirmed the findings in preschoolers, elementary school children and young teens.

The effects of behavioral parent training are larger in specific domains, such as compliance with parental requests, rule-following, defiant/aggressive behavior, and parenting skills (Anastopoulos et al. 1993), than on specific symptoms of ADHD (MTA Cooperative Group 1999, 2004; Daly et al. 2007).

Parent training has developed further into addressing issues such as beliefs, emotions and wider social issues along with issues that hinder the effectiveness of parents such as poor self-esteem, low mood, social isolation and marital difficulties.

Parent training programs are structured and follow a set curriculum over several weeks. They are mainly conducted in groups, but can be modified for individual treatments. An example of a recognized program is: The Incredible Years by Carolyn Webster-Stratton. See below for a description of some approaches to behavioral therapy. These programs target different age groups.

- **Examples of behavior therapy approaches**

<u>Tangible rewards</u>

Training of parents and teachers in the use of tangible rewards is effective in increasing desired behaviors. Parents can use token systems, behavior charts, or immediate rewards such as extra time for recreational and leisure activities, or the mean to obtain items that the young person likes or appreciates.

Schemes using "tokens" (such as stars, chips, marbles and so on) may, for little children, be rewarding, whereas for older children tokens may be exchanged for items of value to them as gifts.

<u>Response cost or negative consequences</u>

Using a point or token system is one in which negative behaviors result in the loss of points or tokens. Training parents and teachers to use response cost is effective in reducing undesired behavior. Penalties may increase based on severity of behavior.

<u>Time out</u>

Place the child away from the attention of others for a set period of time.

<u>Parent monitoring</u>

Give parents a structured way to monitor their child's behavior. It can be an informal measure, such as daily homework log, or a formal measure using a scale.

<u>Praise</u>

Praise can be achieved verbally and should be honest, not over flattering, specific and immediate.

In teens, according to Barkley, "Encourage parents to set aside 15 min a few times a week to pay attention to their adolescent" and praise their good behavior.

- **Cognitive therapy (CBT)**
  Although CBT is not demonstrated as efficacious in children who have ADHD, there are reasons to continue to do more research in adolescents who have ADHD. For example, CBT generally is more effective in adolescents relative to preadolescents (Holmbeck et al. 2003). Future research should consider the extent to which CBT is effective for adolescents who have ADHD.
- **Peer based intervention and social skills training**
  Peers rated children with ADHD as lower on social preference, higher on social impact, less well liked, and more often in the rejected social status category. Children with ADHD have fewer dyadic friendships. Children with ADHD tend to be more impulsive, argumentative, and aggressive than their typically developing peers, and are often rejected by their peers (Hodgens et al. 2000; Hoza et al. 2005). There is evidence that combining social skills interventions with behavior management program and parent training does improve ADHD children's behavior toward their peers (Sheridan et al. 1996).
  Suggested approaches for social skills training include:
  - systematic teaching of social skills,
  - social problem solving,
  - teaching other behavioral skills often considered important by children, such as sports skills and board game rules,
  - decreasing undesirable and antisocial behaviors, such as anger,
  - developing a close friendship.

  There are several settings for providing these interventions to children, including groups in office clinics, classrooms, small groups at school and summer camps (Jacobs 2005).

  Some authors have argued that in addition to social skills training, problem solving approaches are also required. They have been developed and are concerned with the child and young person's ability to self-regulate (the capacity of the child and young person to initiate, delay, modify or modulate the amount, or intensity, of a thought, emotion, behavior or psychological response), cope with stress, and learn relaxation techniques (Compas 2002).
- **Family therapy**
  There are many models of family therapy that are aiming at producing changes in the ways that families function. The central goal of family therapy is to reduce the level of negative emotions, and to address the family's approach to problem solving and conflict resolution.
- **Educational interventions**
  <u>Classroom based behavioral management</u>
  Behavioral classroom interventions generally involve regular consultation with the child's teacher regarding the use of behavior modification strategies. Consultation usually begins with psychoeducation about ADHD and identification of specific target behaviors, based upon a functional assessment of behavior (i.e., examination of antecedents, behaviors, and consequences). Teachers are then instructed regarding the use of specific behavioral techniques, including praise, planned ignoring, effective commands, and time out, as well as the daily report card (DRC), and/or more extensive individualized or classroom-wide contingency

management programs. Behaviorally based classroom interventions appear to be a very effective means of behavior change in children with ADHD in the school setting. However, as cooperation of school professionals is necessary for these interventions, some of the same challenges exist as with home behavioral programs. That is, beneficial treatment effects rely on the consistent use of behavior modification techniques by teachers, who are sometimes resistant or unable to implement such programs as intended (Chronis et al. 2006).

Academic and educational interventions

Individuals with ADHD suffer significant deficits in executive functioning (time management, organization, etc.) which can cause marked impairment at school/college and work. This places the individual with ADHD at a significant disadvantage for completing tasks, projects and tests on time. The following approaches were reviewed by Raggi and Chronis in 2006:

- Peer tutoring: Advantages of this approach include one-to-one individualized instructions, frequent and immediate feedback, active participation of students, and high levels of practicality and acceptability. Peer tutoring can be implemented by teachers in a general education setting with a high level of fidelity using a resource (i.e., peer tutors) that is readily available in the classroom. Parent tutoring procedures may be useful in combination with peer tutoring in the classroom.
- Computer-assisted instruction (CAI): Advantages of CAI include providing immediate feedback and requiring active responding on the part of the student. The CAI approach may be highly desirable for use in classroom because it allows teachers more flexibility and time for individualized instruction, and provides an alternative to traditional instruction that may successfully capture the attention of children with ADHD.
- Task/instructional modifications: Task or instructional modifications involve implementing procedures such as reducing task length, dividing tasks into subunits and setting goals for the child to achieve in shorter time intervals, using increases stimulation of the task (e.g., color or texture), giving explicit instructions, and modifying the delivery or modality of instruction depending on the student's individual learning style (e.g., fast-paced versus slow-paced, visual verses auditory).
- Visual versus auditory presentation of material: As children with ADHD have been theorized to have difficulties in the internalization of speech (i.e., working memory deficits), having them respond orally may allow for a greater integration and retention of material than when they must learn information silently.
- Adding structure to a task: Adding structure to a task may increase the saliency of appropriate responses in children with ADHD, thereby lessening the need for self-produced stimulation (Barkley 2005). Head phones and voice dictation have been used as well.
- Choice making: Choice making allows the child a certain level of individual decision-making and personal control over the nature of the task. This consists of allowing the child to select academic tasks or materials from a number of pertinent and structured alternatives. This technique may be

beneficial not only in increasing task performances and productivity, but also in improving social relatedness.
  - Self-monitoring: Self-monitoring and self-reinforcement procedures are widely used and are emerging as effective tools in improving social and academic behavior in the classroom setting in general.
  - Strategy training: Strategy training involves teaching and transferring a specific skill to children that they can implement in an academic situation to improve their performance.
  - Homework-focused interventions: This approach may be particularly useful for children and adolescents with ADHD, who, due to forgetfulness, lack of organization, and impulsivity in conveying information, may often not bring homework materials home or write down homework assignments, and may convey inaccurate information about projects and assignments to parents. Teaching parents to structure the homework process, use goal setting, and consult with school staff are intervention approaches that have been tested and found effective for use with general populations of students with academic problems.
  - Classroom interventions: Examples include:
    - seating arrangements (front or back of class, standing desk, ability to get up and move during class),
    - modified testing (oral testing, more time, testing in a quiet environment), and
    - for children with disabilities, special education classes.

12.4 Predictors of Response to Psychosocial Treatment

A number of published articles (several from the MTA Cooperative Group) have investigated potential mediators and moderators of ADHD treatment effects, including:

- Child comorbidity: It has been argued that behavior modification is a component of effective treatment for several childhood disorders (e.g. ODD, CD, anxiety, depression, autism), and when based on a functional analysis of problematic behaviors, can effectively address most co-occurring disorders.
- Parental psychopathology: This is considered a significant barrier to good response to psychosocial treatment, particularly parent training. Comprehensive treatments for ADHD may benefit from adjunctive treatment components addressing parental psychopathology.
- Parental cognitions and belief: The findings from the MTA study suggested that negative parental cognitions about themselves, their ADHD children, and their parenting were associated with poorer response to behavioral, pharmacological, and combined treatments for ADHD.
- Socioeconomic status (SES): Low SES has been shown to contribute to poor compliance with, and poor outcome, following parent training for noncompliant children.

Race or ethnicity: Differences in cultural norms, expectations about children and parenting, or attitudes regarding mental health, may influence treatment attainment, compliance or outcomes.

12.5 Overview – Adults

Pharmacologic studies show that stimulant medication is moderately effective in treating adult ADHD, but residual symptoms are common, supporting the need for adjunctive behavioral interventions (Wilens et al. 2002). The psychological treatment in adults may start to address feelings of helplessness and low self-esteem that accompany ADHD in some cases. Individuals who have not received their diagnosis until adulthood will require psychological support as they often appear to undergo a process of acceptance and understanding associated with their late diagnosis (Young and Gudjonsson 2008). Furthermore, CBT has a strong evidence base for many of the comorbid disorders associated with ADHD. A growing body of empirical evidence supports structured, skills-based psychosocial treatment for ADHD in adults as a valuable adjunctive treatment to stimulate medications. Both individual and group-based treatment appear to be valuable (Krouse et al. 2008). Psychosocial interventions can include cognitive behavioral therapy (CBT), self-management skills training, environmental restructuring, psychoeducation, individual psychotherapy, family therapy, marital or couple therapy, vocational counseling, and ADHD coaching (Davidson 2008).

Australian Draft Guidelines – Recommendations:

(Please refer to the copyright permission given at the beginning of the book.)

- *For adults whose ADHD has been stabilized on medication, a course of either group or individual cognitive behavioral therapy (CBT) could be considered to improve ADHD symptoms further and assist with daily function in areas such as organizational skills, self-esteem and social skills.*
- *Psychoeducation, counseling, psychotherapy or coaching may benefit some adults with ADHD.*
- *Consideration of the use of psychosocial interventions should take into account availability and the individual's resources and capacity to adhere to the program.*

12.6 Psychosocial Interventions – Adults

- **Cognitive Behavioral Therapy (CBT)**

  CBT interventions may be used with adults to help them develop strategies and learn practical techniques to reduce the impact of their ADHD symptoms on their functioning. For example, time awareness, facilitation of task initiation and completion by dividing it in to small parts, contingent self-reward, scheduling and prioritizing, maintaining motivation by visualizing long term reward. Traditional CBT methods should also target depression and anxiety, because of mood and anxiety problems that interfere with efficient self-management.

Treatment can be offered on a group or individual basis, vary in duration and may be provided only as brief intensive treatments, such as brief solution-focused therapy or weekly treatment over a few months.

An individualized CBT intervention was develop for adult ADHD that included psychoeducation about ADHD; skills training in organization, planning and maximizing attention (e.g., breaking down large tasks into smaller components); and cognitive restructuring to maximize adaptive thinking and reduce distractions (Safren et al. 2005).

CBT approaches may be particularly useful for adults with ADHD because the structured nature of the sessions allow the patient and the therapist to follow a specific agenda relevant to the patient's goals, and therefore, stay on target with the goals of the treatment (Krouse et al. 2008). Research is currently being conducted by Dr. Lilly Hechtman and her team at McGill University around CBT in adults. The initial results have been promising.

- **Coaching**
  Coaching is aimed at helping people with ADHD to identify strengths, negotiate problems, and work on specific goals. Regular contact, and the formation of partnership with the coach, provide a supportive framework that help to build confidence in taking on specific tasks. There are no rigorous clinical trials demonstrating that coaching of any type is an effective intervention in the treatment of adults with ADHD. Goldstein (2005) expressed his concern that "professionals from diverse mental health, business, and educational backgrounds" promote coaching as a service they offer without enough support of scientific studies (Goldstein 2005; Kubik 2010).
- **Psychoeducation**
  Psychoeducation is an integral part of treatment of ADHD. Some authors also suggested that bibliotherapy can be useful in answering questions from patients and their families (M. D. Weiss and Weiss 2004). After receiving a diagnosis, education about the effects of ADHD is generally agreed on as a starting point for ADHD psychosocial treatment (Ramsay and Rostain 2007). Adults with ADHD can learn more about the disorder and how it affects them specifically, which can aid in their ability to cope with the disorder and the development of individualized treatment plans (Murphy 2005; Davidson 2008).
- **Vocational and Academic testing and support**
  Patients with ADHD may benefit from vocational testing. Some specific accommodations might be required in certain jobs. Symptoms of ADHD can significantly impair workplace performance. Impulsivity, inattention, disorganization, careless mistakes, poor time management, and inconsistency can all lead to employment difficulties. Vocational counseling can help alleviate occupational difficulties by identifying strengths and limitations and by matching adults to jobs that are well suited for them (Barkley 2006; Weiss and Weiss 2004). Academic remediation and specialized educational placement might also be helpful.
- **Psychotherapy**
  Individual psychotherapy generally comprises of a number of components, including psychoeducation, the setting of treatment goals and establishment of

strategies to meet those goals, problem solving, and dealing with the comorbid problems that often accompany ADHD (Barkley 2006; Murphy 2005). Family and marital or couples therapy from an ADHD perspective can be very helpful to address the dysfunction and the disruption to the routine tasks of daily living (Davidson 2008).

General References and Recommended Readings – Children/Adolescents

Anastopoulos AD, Shelton TL, DuPaul GJ, Guevremont DC (1993) Parent training for attention-deficit hyperactivity disorder: its impact on parent functioning. J Abnorm Child Psychol 21(5):581–596

Antshel KM, Barkley R (2008) Psychosocial interventions in attention deficit hyperactivity disorder. Child Adolesc Psychiatr Clin N Am 17(2):421–437

Chronis AM, Chacko A, Fabiano GA, Wymbs BT, Pelham WE Jr (2004) Enhancements to the behavioral parent training paradigm for families of children with ADHD: review and future directions. Clin Child Fam Psychol Rev 7(1):1–27

Chronis AM, Jones HA, Raggi VL (2006) Evidence-based psychosocial treatments for children and adolescents with attention-deficit/hyperactivity disorder. Clin Psychol Rev 26(4):486–502

Compas BE, Benson M, Boyer M, et al (2002) Problem-solving and problem-solving therapies. In: Rutter M, Taylor E (eds) Child and Adolescent Psychiatry, 4th edn. Blackwell, Oxford, pp 938–948

Daly BP, Creed T, Xanthopoulos M et al (2007) Psychosocial treatments for children with attention deficit/hyperactivity disorder. Neuropsychol Rev 17:73–89

Davidson M (2008) ADHD in adults: a review of the literature. J Att Disord 11:628

Dupaul GJ, Eckert TL (1997) The effects of school-based interventions for attention deficit hyperactivity disorder: a meta-analysis. Sch Psychol Rev 26:5–27

Evans SW, Serpell ZM, Schultz BK et al (2007) Cumulative benefits of secondary school-based treatment of students with attention deficit hyperactivity disorder. Sch Psychol Rev 36:256–273

Hodgens JB, Cole J, Boldizar J (2000) Peer-based differences among boys with ADHD. J Clin Child Psychol 29(3):443–452

Holmbeck GE, Greenley RN, Franks EA (2003) Developmental issues and consideration in research and practice. In: Kazdin A, Weisz JR (eds) Evidence-based psychotherapies for children and adolescents. Guilford Press, New York, pp 21–401

Hoza B, Gerdes AC, Mrug S et al (2005) Peer-assessed outcomes in the multimodal treatment study of children with attention deficit hyperactivity disorder. J Clin Child Adolesc Psychol 34:74–86

Jacobs B (2005) Queensland children at risk: the overdiagnosis of "ADHD" and the overuse of stimulant medication. Youth Affairs Network of Queensland, West End. Available at http:// www.yang,org.au

Jensen PS, Arnold LE, Swanson JM et al (2007) 3-year follow up of the NIMH MTA study. J Am Acad Child Adolesc Psychiatry 46:989–1002

Jones K, Daley D, Hutchings J et al (2007) Efficacy of the incredible years basic parent training programme as an early intervention for children with conduct problems and ADHD. Child Care Health Dev 33:749–756

Jurbergs N, Palcic J, Kelley ML (2007) School/home notes with and without response cost: increasing attention and academic performance in low-income children with attention-deficit hyperactivity disorder. Sch Psychol Q 22:358–379

Kaiser NM, Hoza B, Hurt EA (2008) Multimodal treatment for childhood attention deficit/hyperactivity disorder. Expert Rev Neurother 8(10):1573–1583

MTA Cooperative Group (1999) A 14-month randomized clinical trial of treatment strategies for attention-deficit/hyperactivity disorder. The MTA Cooperative Group. Multimodal Treatment Study of Children with ADHD. Arch Gen Psychiatry 56(12):1073–1086

MTA Cooperative Group (2004) The National Institute for Mental Health Multimodal Treatment Study of ADHD follow up: 24 month outcomes of treatment strategies for attention deficit/hyperactivity disorder. Pediatrics 113:754–761
Murphy K (2005) Psychosocial treatments for ADHD in teens and adults: a practice-friendly review. J Clin Psychol 61(5):607–619
Pelham WE, Fabiano GA (2008) Evidence-based psychosocial treatments for attention-deficit/hyperactivity disorder. J Clin Child Adolesc Psychol 37:184–214
Pfiffner LJ, Mikami AY, Huang-Pollock C et al (2007) A randomized, controlled trial of integrated home-school behavioral treatment for ADHD, predominantly inattentive type. J Am Acad Child Adolesc Psychiatry 46:1041–1050
Rader R, McCauley L, Callen EC (2009) Current strategies in the diagnosis and treatment of childhood attention deficit/hyperactivity disorder. Am Fam Physician 79(8):657–665
Raggi VL, Chronis AM (2006) Interventions to address the academic impairment of children and adolescents with ADHD. Clin Child Family Psychol Rev 9:85–111
Sheridan SM, Dee CC, Morgan JC, McCormick ME, Walker D (1996) A multimethod intervention for social skills deficits in children with ADHD and their parents. School Psychology Review, 25:57–76
Van den Hoofdakker BJ, van der Veen-Mulders L, System S et al (2007) Effectiveness of behavioral parent training for children with ADHD in routine clinical practice: a randomized controlled study. J Am Acad Child Adolesc Psychiatry 46:1263–1271
Webster-Stratton C (2001) The incredible years: parents, teachers, and children training series. In: Pfeiffer SI, Reddy LA (eds) Innovative mental health interventions for children: programs that work. Haworth Press, Binghamton, pp 31–45
Wells KC, Chi TC, Hinshaw SP, Epstein JN, Pfiffner L, Nebel-Schwalm M et al (2006) Treatment-related changes in objectively measured parenting behaviors in the multimodal treatment study of children with attention-deficit/hyperactivity disorder. J Consult Clin Psychol 74(4):649
Young S, Gudjonsson GH (2008) Growing out of ADHD the relationship between functioning and symptoms. J Atten Disord 12(2):162–169

General References and Recommended Readings – Adults and General

Barkley RA (2005) Attention deficit hyperactivity disorder: ADHD handbook for diagnostic and treatment, 2nd edn. Guilford Press, New York
Barkley RA (2006) Attention deficit hyperactivity disorder: a handbook for diagnosis and treatment, 3rd edn. Guilford Press, New York
Barkley RA, Fischer M, Smallish L, Fletcher K (2002) The persistence of attention deficit/hyperactivity disorder into young adulthood as a function of reporting source and definition of the disorder. J Abnorm Psychol 111:279–289
Goldstein SA (2005) Coaching as a treatment for ADHD. Editorial. J Atten Disord 9:379–381
Goodman DW (2007) The consequences of attention deficit/hyperactivity disorder in adults. J Psychiatr Pract 13(5):318–327. Review
Knight LA, Rooney M, Chronis-Tuscano A (2008) Psychosocial treatments for attention deficit/hyperactivity disorder. Curr Psychiatr Rep 10(5):412–418. Review
Krouse LE, Cooper-Vince C, Sprich S, Safren SA (2008) Recent developments in the psychosocial treatment of adults ADHD. Expert Rev Neurother 8(10):1537–1548. Review
Kubik JA (2010) Efficacy of ADHD coaching for adults with ADHD. J Atten Disord 13(5):442–453
Ramsay JR, Rostain AL (2007) Psychosocial treatments for attention-deficit/hyperactivity disorder in adults: current evidence and future directions. Prof Psychol Res Pract 38:338–346

Safren SA, Otto MW, Sprich W et al (2005) Cognitive-behavioral therapy for ADHD in medication-treated adults with continued symptoms. Behav Res Ther 43(7):831–842

Solanto MV, Marks DJ, Mitchell KJ et al (2008) Development of a new psychosocial treatment for adult ADHD. J Atten Disord 11:728–736

Weiss MD, Weiss JR (2004) A guide to the treatment of adults with ADHD. J Clin Psychiatry 65(3):23–37

Wilens TE, Biederman J, Spencer TJ (2002) Attention deficit/hyperactivity disorder across the lifespan. Annu Rev Med 53:113–131

ADHD Guidelines Available on the Internet

American Psychological Association: http://www.apa.org/topics/adhd/index.aspx

Australian ADHD Draft Guidelines: http://www.nhmrc.gov.au/guidelines/publications/ch54

Canadian ADHD Guidelines: http://www.caddra.ca/cms4/

National Institute for Health and Clinical Excellence (NICE): http://publications.nice.org.uk/attention-deficit-hyperactivity-disorder-cg72

Scottish ADHD Guidelines: http://www.sign.ac.uk/guidelines/fulltext/112/index.html

13 Follow-Up of Patients with ADHD

According to Australian Draft Guidelines (2009) the following recommendations were made:

- Individuals on medication for ADHD should be monitored by their treating physician for medication effectiveness and side effects. This should occur frequently in the early phase of treatment, and thereafter at intervals of 3–6 months.
- Consider using standard symptom and side effect rating scales throughout the course of treatment as an adjunct to clinical assessment for people with ADHD.
- Use a functional scale to follow improvement in functional impairment. An example would be the Weiss Functional Impairment Scale.
- Monitoring should include reports from caregivers, partners, and/or teachers (as applicable). Brief parent and teacher behavior rating scales can also contribute to monitoring of behavior or performance at home or school.
- Monitoring at each visit should include height, weight and growth in children and adolescents. Monitor also for psychiatric disturbance, heart rate and blood pressure in all age groups.
- Monitor for medication misuse or diversion, and substance use.
- In adults, sexual dysfunction (that is erectile and ejaculatory dysfunction or dysmenorrhea) should be monitored as potential side effects of Atomoxetine.
- Monitor for other side effects such as anxiety, tics, seizure, insomnia, headaches, and gastrointestinal effects.
- Sometimes, trials off medication can be helpful to evaluate whether the medication is still clinically indicated.

ADHD Guidelines Available on the Internet

American Psychological Association: http://www.apa.org/topics/adhd/index.aspx
Australian ADHD Draft Guidelines: http://www.nhmrc.gov.au/guidelines/publications/ch54
Canadian ADHD Guidelines: http://www.caddra.ca/cms4/
National Institute for Health and Clinical Excellence (NICE): http://publications.nice.org.uk/attention-deficit-hyperactivity-disorder-cg72
Scottish ADHD Guidelines: http://www.sign.ac.uk/guidelines/fulltext/112/index.html

J. Sadek, *A Clinician's Guide to ADHD*,
DOI 10.1007/978-3-319-02359-5_13,

Books for the Public

14

Title	Author	ISBN
Delivered from Distraction	**Hallowell and Ratey**	978-0-345-44231-4
Driven to Distraction	**Edward Hallowell and John Ratey**	9780307743152
Is It You, Me or the Adult ADD	**Gina Pera**	978-0-9815487-0-8
Understand Your Brain – Get More Done	**Ari Tuckman**	978-1-886941-39-7
10 Simple Solutions to Adult ADHD	**Stephanie Moulton Sarkis**	978-1572244344
You Mean I'm Not Lazy, Stupid or Crazy?	**Kate Kelly and Peggy Ramundo**	978-0684815312
ADD Friendly Ways to Organize Your Life	**Judith Kobler Kathleen Nadeau**	978-1583913581
Women with Attention Deficit Disorder	**Sari Solden**	978-1887424974
Spark	**Dr. John Ratey**	978-0316113502
The ADHD Effect on Marriage	**Melissa Orlov**	978-1886941977
The Disorganized Mind: Coaching Your ADHD Brain to Take Control of Your Time, Tasks, and Talents	**Nancy A. Ratey**	978-0312355340
Taking Change of Adult ADHD	**Russell Barkley**	978-1606233382
Getting Paid to Pay Attention – Why Your Business Suffers from ADD and How to Fix It	**Marilyn Strong**	978-0921470021
The Complete Idiot's Guide to Adult ADHD	**Eileen Bailey and Donald Haupt, M.D.**	978-1615640065
ADD Stole My Car Keys	**Rick Green and Umesh Jain**	978-0986624025

J. Sadek, *A Clinician's Guide to ADHD*,
DOI 10.1007/978-3-319-02359-5_14, © Springer International Publishing Switzerland 2014

15 List of Scales – Children

- **Behavior Assessment System for Children (BASC):** This scale addresses externalizing and internalizing problems, as well as school problems. It has a behavioral symptoms index and adaptive skills index. (broad band).
- **Child Behavior Checklist (CBCL):** There are two forms of this scale, one is a parent completed and the other is teacher completed (TRF). It is available at www.aseba.org/index.html. (broad band).
- **Academic Performance Rating Scale (APRS):** The APRS is a 19 item scale for determining a child's academic productivity and accuracy in grades 1–6 that has six scale points; construct, concurrent and discriminant validity data, as well as norms (n = 247) available (Barkley 1990).
- **ADHD Rating Scale-IV:** The ADHD Rating Scale-IV is an 18 item scale using DSM-IV criteria (DuPaul et al. 2003). It can be completed by either parents (home form) or teachers (school form).
- **Brown ADD Rating Scales (BADDS):** It was first published in self-reporting format in 1996 for adolescents. It focused on the inattention and executive dysfunction not always apparent to observers. In the revised format different scales have been developed for different age groups, such as 3–7, 8–12, and 12–18 years of age, thus focusing on the symptoms of ADHD through the different development stages. Self-report format is available from age 8 and up, parent and teacher scales are available for all ages. The tools are available at: www.drthomasebrown.com/assess_tools/index.html.

  BADDS includes five clinically derived subscales or "clusters": (1) Organizing, Prioritizing and Activating to Work; (2) Focusing, Sustaining, and Shifting Attention to Tasks; (3) Regulating Alertness, Sustaining Effort, and Processing Speed; (4) Managing Frustration and Modulating Emotions; and (5) Utilizing Working Memory and Accessing Recall.
- **Conners Rating Scale (Revised):** CPRS-R is a parent and adolescent self-report version (Conners 1997); for teachers Conners Teacher Rating Scale – Revised (CTRS-R) (Conners 1997); for adolescents Conners Wells Adolescent Self-Report Scale (Conners and Wells 1997) (broad band).

J. Sadek, *A Clinician's Guide to ADHD*,
DOI 10.1007/978-3-319-02359-5_15,

- **Conners Rating Scale Revised (CRS-R):** This is a parent, teacher and adolescent self-reporting scale, each being available in long and short format. There are also three screening tools that give the option of administering a 12 item ADHD Index or an 18 item Symptoms Checklist (DSM-IV), or both. This is considered a broad band.
- **Copeland Symptom Checklist for Attention Deficit Disorders – Child and Adolescent Versions:** This checklist designed in 1987 addresses ten key areas, including: emotional difficulties, peer relationships, family interaction issues, maturity level, distractibility, activity level, impulsivity, degree of compliance, attention-seeking behaviors, and cognitive and visual-motor achievement.
- **Home Situations Questionnaire – Revised (HSQ-R), School Situations Questionnaire – Revised (SSQ-R):** The HSQ-R is a 14 item scale designed for parent reporting to assess specific problems with attention and concentration across a variety of home and public situations that most commonly occur day to day. It takes about 5 min to complete and is used with ages 4–11.

  The teacher version, SSQ-R is a 12 item tool that identifies frequency and severity of the child's behavioral problems at school. The age range for this format is also 4–11 and takes 5 min to complete (Barkley 1990).
- **Inattention/Overactivity with Aggression (IOWA) Conners Rating Scale:** The IOWA Conners is a ten item scale developed to rate inattention/overactivity ratings and separate them from oppositional defiance. This instrument was one of the first rating scales developed to evaluate children and adolescents with ADHD.
- **Swanson, Nolan and Pelham (SNAP-IV):** The SNAP-IV (Forness 1992) is a 26 item scale that reflects DSM-III criteria for ADHD. It also screens for other DSM diagnoses. The SNAP-IV-Revised (SNAP-IV-R) (using DSM-IV criteria) is and 90 item scale for use with children ages 6–18 and takes about 10 min to administer. It includes symptoms of oppositional defiant disorder (ODD) and aggression. It is available at www.caddra.ca.
- **SKAMP (Swanson, Kotkin, Agler, M-Flynn and Pelham):** The SKAMP (Wigal et al. 1998) is a ten item scale that measures impairment of functioning at home and at school. Separate subscales measure the severity of impairment of inattention.
- **Vanderbilt ADHD Scale:** This is a diagnostic tool for parents and teachers that rates 35 symptoms and eight performance items measuring ADHD symptoms and common comorbid conditions (Wolraich et al. 2003). The parent version contains all 18 ADHD symptoms, with items assessing comorbid conditions and performance. The Vanderbilt Assessment Scale has two components: symptoms assessment and an assessment of impairment of performance at home, school, and other social settings. This rating scale is used by professionals to screen for ADHD, oppositional defiant disorder, conduct disorder, anxiety and depression in children. The parent rating scale version contains 55 items, while the teacher version has 43 items and focuses on behavior an observations at school. Each takes about 10 min to complete, is free on line and is suitable for ages 6–12.

Other tests:

- **Intelligence tests** are not required to diagnose ADHD but they can be used in some cases during the general assessment. Examples are the **Wechsler Intelligence Scale for Children (WISC) and Stanford-Binet test**.
- **Achievement tests** are also not required to diagnose ADHD but are designed to measure a child's current level of functioning with regard to specific academic subjects, such as reading, writing, and math. They may also test knowledge and skills. Examples are **Woodcock-Johnson III, Wechsler Individual Achievement Test (WIAT), Wide Range Achievement Test (WRAT)**.
- **Attention tests** may also be useful. There is a wide variety to choose from. Examples are the **Conners CPT II Continuous Performance Test II (Version 5 for Windows), Integrated Visual and Auditory Continuous Performance Test (IVA), Tests for Variable Attention (TOVA)**.
- **Executive functioning** that includes problem solving abilities (i.e., reasoning, planning, and organization), flexibility in thinking, and the ability to integrate feedback from others and abstract can also be tested. Examples include the **Wisconsin Card Sort Test (WCST)**. This test is not a mandatory part of ADHD assessment.

NB: AACAP Practice parameter for the Assessment and Treatment of Children and Adolescents with ADHD compiled a list of scales that is very useful.

NB: Some free scales available at www.caddra.ca

General References and Recommended Readings

AACAP. Practice parameter for the assessment and treatment of children and adolescents with ADHD. J Am Acad Child Adolesc Psychiatry. 2007;46(7):894–921

Achenbach TM (1991) Manual for the child behavior checklist. University of Vermont, Department of Psychiatry, Burlington

Barkley RA, Murphy KR (1998) Attention-deficit/hyperactivity disorder: a clinical workbook, 2nd edn. Guilford Press, New York

Barkley RA, DuPaul GJ, McMurray MB (1990) Comprehensive evaluation of attention deficit disorder with and without hyperactivity as defined by research criteria. J Consult Clin Psychol 58(6):775–789

Conners CK (1997) Conners' rating scales—revised user's manual. Multi Health Systems, Inc., North Tonawanda

Conners CK, Wells KC, Parker JDA et al (1997) A new self-report scale for assessment of adolescent psychopathology: factor structure, reliability, validity, and diagnostic sensitivity. Journal of Abnormal Child Psychology 25:487–497

DuPaul GJ (1991) Parent and teacher ratings of ADHD symptoms: psychometric properties in a community-based sample. J Clin Child Psychol 20(3):245–253

DuPaul GJ, Stoner G (2003) ADHD in the schools: assessment and intervention strategies. Guildford Press, New York

Forness, Youpa, Hanna, Cantwell, Swanson (1992) Classroom instructional characteristics in attention deficit hyperactivity disorder: Comparison of pure and mixed subgroups. Behavioral Disorders 17:115–125

Kamphaus RW, Reynolds CR (1998) BASC monitor for ADHD: manual and software guide. American Guidance Service, Circle Pines

Rader R, McCauley L, Callen EC (2009) Current strategies in the diagnosis and treatment of childhood attention-deficit/hyperactivity disorder. Am Fam Physician 79(8):657–665. Review

Reynolds CR, Kamphaus RW (1992) BASC: behavior assessment system for children: manual. American Guidance Service, Inc., Circle Pines
Taylor A et al (2011) Scales for the identification of adults with ADHD: a systematic review. Res Dev Disabil 32(3):924–938
Ullmann RK, Sleator EK, Sprague RL (1984) A new rating scale for diagnosis and monitoring of ADD children. Psychopharmacol Bull 20(1):160–164
Wigal T, Swanson JM, Douglas VI et al (1998) Effect of reinforcement on facial responsivity and persistence in children with attention-deficit hyperactivity disorder. Behavior Modification 22:143–166
Wolraich ML, Lambert W, Doffing MA, Bickman L, Simmons T, Worley K (2003) Psychometric properties of the Vanderbilt ADHD diagnostic parent rating scale in a referred population. J Pediatr Psychol 28(8):559–568

16 List of Scales – Adults

- **Adult Self Report Scale (ASRS):** This is based on self-report of current symptoms and has long version 18 items and short version six items. Symptom frequency is based on a five point Likert scale (0–4). The six items with the most stable psychometric properties were chosen for the short ASRS.
- **Adult Rating Scale (ARS):** This is based on self and informant report of childhood and current symptoms with 25 items using Likert scale (0–3). The items are derived from the DSM-III-R criteria, and is of similar format to the children's version of this scale.
- **ADHD Rating Scale (ADHD-RS):** This is based on self and informant report of childhood and current symptoms. This is a self-reporting scale with a long (18 items – 9 inattention, 9 hyperactivity) and short version (six items) of current symptoms using a Likert scale (0–3). Criteria used: DSM-IV.
- **Attention Deficit Scales for Adults (ADSA):** This is a self-reporting scale of current symptoms with 54 items using a five point rating (1–5). Answers are recorded on an answer sheet. This scale was developed based on clinical experience and is divided into nine subscales: attention, interpersonal, disorganization, co-ordination, academic theme, emotive, long term, childhood and negative social elements. Additionally an inconsistency index is included.
- **Adult Problems Questionnaire (APQ):** This is a self-reporting scale of current symptoms with 43 items (score range 0–3) that includes the common symptoms of ADHD adults. The questions are based on the DSM-IV and the Utah criteria.
- **Assessment of Hyperactivity and Attention (AHA):** This is both a self-reporting and informant rating scale of current and childhood symptoms. Eighteen items rate based on DSM-IV criteria. Here answers are given with a "yes" or "no" reply, and two subscales are covered including inattention and hyperactivity.
- **Brown Attention Deficit Disorder Scales (BADDS):** This 40 item self-reporting scale of current symptoms is divided into five subscales those being organization/work, attention, energy/effort, mood and memory. A scoring sheet is used for answering. Items are based on DSM-IV criteria, as well as based on the author's clinical observations and several studies.

J. Sadek, *A Clinician's Guide to ADHD*,

DOI 10.1007/978-3-319-02359-5_16,

- **Caterino Scale:** Used for both self- or informant reporting, this 18 item scale focuses on adult and childhood symptoms. It is based on DSM-IV criteria and the psychologist chosen behaviors that reflect DSM-IV. It has no cut off score
- **Current Symptoms Scale (CSS):** Another self-reporting scale with two subscales of nine items each on inattention and hyperactivity/impulsivity. Rating on a 0–3 Likert scale, the items are specifically from the DSM-IV 'A' criteria. It has been used for retrospective childhood symptom report.
- **Conners Adult ADHD Rating Scale (CAARS):** There is both a long and short version of this rating scale (66 long, 26 short) and can be completed by the patient or someone else reporting current symptoms. This scale was developed from the children's version and the Utah criteria of nine domains. T scores between 50 and 65 are considered borderline and require interpretation by trained clinician.
- **Symptom Inventory (SI):** An 18 scale self-report of current symptoms broken down into two subscales: inattention and hyperactivity/impulsivity. This was developed for use in the developers' clinic based on the DSM-IV criteria.
- **Wender Utah ADHD Rating Scale (WURS):** The WURS includes a long (61 item) and short (25 item) self-reporting scale that includes current and childhood symptoms. Items were taken from Wender's "Minimal Brain Dysfunction in Children". The short version can also be reported by other than patient informant. It has robust psychometric properties. Symptom frequency is based on a five point Likert scale (0–4).
- **Young Adults Questionnaire (YAQ):** This is a 112 item scale for self-reporting of childhood symptoms. There are four subscales (ADHD symptoms, emotional delinquency and social environments). This scale was developed based on a literature review of ADHD symptoms and co-morbid factors.
- **Young Adult Rating Scale (YARS):** Here 24 items mostly all based on DSM-Iv criteria report an individual's current symptoms, including those experienced during college.

Snap Scale – Children

17

17.1 The SNAP-IV Teacher and Parent Rating Scale

James M. Swanson, PH.D., University of California, Irvine, CA 92715

Name: ______________________________ Gender: __________

Age: _______ Grade: ______

Ethnicity (circle one which best applies):

African-American Asian Caucasian Hispanic Other _____________

For each item, check the column which best describes this child:	Not at all	Just a little	Quite a bit	Very much
1. Often fails to give close attention to details or makes careless mistakes in schoolwork or tasks				
2. Often has difficulty sustaining attention tasks or play activities				
3. Often does not seem ta listen when spoken to directly				
4. Often does not follow through on instructions and fails to finish schoolwork, chores or duties				
5. Often has difficulty organizing tasks and activities				
6. Often avoids, dislikes, or reluctantly engages in tasks requiring sustained mental effort				
7. Often loses things necessary for activities (e.g., toys, school assignments, pencils, or books)				
8. Often is distracted by extraneous stimuli				
9. Often is forgetful in daily activities				
10. Often has difficulty maintaining alertness, orienting to requests, or executing directions				
11. Often fidgets with hands or feet or squirms in seat				
12. Often leaves seat in classroom or in other situations in which remaining seated is expected				
13. Often runs about or climbs excessively in situation in which it is inappropriate				
14. Often has difficulty playing or engaging in leisure activities quietly				

J. Sadek, *A Clinician's Guide to ADHD*,
DOI 10.1007/978-3-319-02359-5_17, © Springer International Publishing Switzerland 2014

For each item, check the column which best describes this child:	Not at all	Just a little	Quite a bit	Very much
15. Often is "on the go" or often acts as if "driven by a motor"				
16. Often talks excessively				
17. Often blurts out answers before questions have been completed				
18. Often has difficulty awaiting turn				
19. Often interrupts or intrudes on others (e.g., buts into conversations/games)				
20. Often has difficulty sitting still, being quiet, or inhibiting impulses in the classroom or at home				
21. Often loses temper				
22. Often argues with adults				
23. Often actively defies or refuses adult requests or rules				
24. Often deliberately does things that annoy other people				
25. Often blames others for his or her mistakes or misbehavior				
26. Often touchy or easily annoyed by others				
27. Often is angry and resentful				
28. Often is spiteful or vindictive				
29. Often is quarrelsome				
30. Often is negative, defiant, disobedient, or hostile toward authority figures				
31. Often makes noises (e.g., humming or odd sounds)				
32. Often is excitable, impulsive				
33. Often cries easily				
34. Often is uncooperative				
35. Often acts "smart"				
36. Often is restless or overactive				
37. Often disturbs other children				
38. Often changes mood quickly and drastically				
39. Often easily frustrated if demands are not met immediately				
40. Often teases other children and interferes with their activities				
41. Often is aggressive to other children (e.g., picks fights or bullies)				
42. Often destructive with property of others (e.g., vandalism)				
43. Often deceitful (e.g., steals, lies, forges, copies the work of others, or "cons" others)				
44. Often and seriously violates rules (e.g., is truant, runs away, or completely ignores class rules)				
45. Has persistent pattern of violating the basic rights of others or major societal norms				
46. Has episodes of failure to resist aggressive impulses (to assault others or to destroy property)				
47. Has motor or verbal tics (sudden, rapid, recurrent, non-rhythmic motor or verbal activity)				

For each item, check the column which best describes this child:	Not at all	Just a little	Quite a bit	Very much
48. Has repetitive motor behavior (e.g., hand waving, body rocking, or picking at skin)				
49. Has obsessions (persistent and intrusive inappropriate ideas, thoughts or impulses)				
50. Has compulsions (repetitive behaviors or mental acts to reduce anxiety or distress)				
51. Often is restless or seems keyed up or on edge				
52. Often is easily fatigued				

17.2 Scoring Instructions for the SNAP-IV-C Rating Scale

The SNAP-IV Rating Scale is a revision of the Swanson, Nolan and Pelham (SNAP) Questionnaire (Swansan et al. 1983). The items from the DSM-IV (1994) criteria for Attention-Deficit/Hyperactivity Disorder (ADHD) are included for the two subsets of symptoms: inattention (items #1–#9) and hyperactivity/impulsivity (items #11–#19). Also, items are included from the DSM-IV criteria for Oppositional Defiant Disorder (items #21–#28) since it often is present in children with ADHD. Items have been added to summarize the Inattention domain (#10) and the Hyperactivity/Impulsivity domain (#20) for ADHD. Two other items were added: an item from DSM-III-R (#29) that was not included in the DSM-IV list of ODD, and an item to summarize the ODD domain (#30).

In addition to the DSM-IV items for ADHD and ODD, the SNAP-IV contains items from the Conners Index Questionnaire (Conners 1968) and the IOWA Conners Questionnaire (Loney and Milich 1985). The IOWA was developed using divergent validity to separate items which measure inattention/over activity (I/O – items #4, #8, #11, #31, #32) from those items which measure aggression/defiance (A/D – items #21, #23, #29, #34, #35). The Conners Index (items #4, #8, #11, #21, #32, #33, #36, #37, #38, #39) was developed by selecting the items which loaded highest on the multiple factors of the Conners Questionnaire, and thus represents a general index of childhood problems.

The SNAP-IV is based on a 0 to 3 rating scale: Not at all=0, Just a little=1, Quite a bit=2, and very much=3. Subscale scores on the SNAP-IV are calculated by summing the scores on the items in the subset and dividing by the number of items in the subset. The score for any subset is expressed as the Average Rating Per Item, as shown for rating on the ADHD-Inattentive (ADHD-I) subset:

	Not at all	Just a little	Quite a bit	Very much	Item score
1. Makes careless mistakes			X		2
2. Can't pay attention				X	3
3. Doesn't listen				X	3
4. Fails to finish work			X		2
5. Disorganized		X			1

	Not at all	Just a little	Quite a bit	Very much	Item score
6. Can't concentrate				X	3
7. Loses things		X			1
8. Distractible				X	3
9. Forgetful	X				0

ADHD-In Total = 18, Average 18/9 = 2.0

A scoring template for the DSM-IV subtypes of ADHD (in and H/Im), for ODD; for the dimensions of the CLAM (I/O and A/D); and for the Coppers Index are presented below:

ADHD-In	ADHD-H/Im	COD	A/D	I/O	Coppers Index
#1 ____	#11 ____	#21 ____	#4 ____	#21 ____	#4 ____
#2 ____	#12 ____	#22 ____	#8 ____	#23 ____	#8 ____
#3 ____	#13 ____	#23 ____	#11 ____	#29 ____	#11 ____
#4 ____	#14 ____	#24 ____	#31 ____	#34 ____	#21 ____
#5 ____	#15 ____	#25 ____	#32 ____	#35 ____	#32 ____
#6 ____	#16 ____	#26 ____			#33 ____
#7 ____	#17 ____	#27 ____			#36 ____
#8 ____	#18 ____	#28 ____			#37 ____
#9 ____	#19 ____				#38 ____
					#39 ____

Total In ·____	H/Im ·____	COD ·____	I/O ·____	A/D ·____	O ·____
Average ·____	·____	·____	·____	·____	·____

C ·____

·____

Temtative 5% cutoff	Teacher	Parent
ADHD-In	2.56	1.78
ADHD-H/Im	1.78	1.44
ADHD-C	2.00	1.67
COD	1.38	1.88

The items on page 2 **[formatting purposes for book = from question 41 and on]** of the SNAP-IV Rating Scale are from other DSM-IV disorders which may overlap with or masquerade as symptoms of ADHD. In some cases, these may be comorbid disorders, but in other cases the presence of one or more of these disorders may be sufficient to exclude a diagnosis of ADHD. The SNAP-IV is not designed to be used in the formal process of diagnosing these non-ADHD disorders, but if symptoms on page 2 **[formatting purposes for book = from question 41 and on]** of the SNAP-IV receive a high "Quite a bit" or "Very much" rating, then an assessment of the implicated non-ADHD disorders may be warranted.

The DSM-IV Manual should be consulted to follow up with an evaluation of these non-ADHD disorders. The DSM Codes and the page numbers in the DSM Manual are specified below to help in the assessment of possible conditions which may exclude or qualify a diagnosis of ADHD. A referral to a psychiatrist or clinical psychologist may be required.

#41–#45	Conduct Disorder	DSM 312.8, p. 85
#46	Intermittent Explosive Disorder	DSM 312.34, p. 609
#47	Tourettes' Disorder	DSM 307.23, p. 103
#48	Stereotypic Movement Disorder	DSM 307.3, p. 121
#49–#50	Obsessive-Compulsive Disorder	DSM 300.3, p. 417
#51–#56	Generalized Anxiety Disorder	DSM 300.02, p. 432
#57	Narcolepsy	DSM 347, p. 562
#58	Histrionic Personality Disorder	DSM 301.50, p. 655
#59	Narcissistic Personality Disorder	DSM 301.81, p. 658
#60	Borderline Personality Disorder	DSM 301.83, p. 650
#61–#65	Manic Episode	DSM 296.00, p. 328
#66–#73	Major Depressive Episode	DSM 296.2, p. 320
#74–#76	Dysthymic Disorder	DSM 300.4, p. 345
#77–#78	Posttraumatic Stress Disorder	DSM 309.81, p.424
#79–#80	Adjustment Disorder	DSM 309, p.623

It is important to note that many disorders may produce impairment in the classroom setting, not just ADHD. Therefore, this rating scale is presented last to be the possible exclusion conditions (#40–#90 of the SNAP-IV) will be considered in addition to the inclusion criteria for ADHD (#1–#40 of the SNAP-IV). Both should be considered before interpreting the SKAMP measure of classroom impairment or attributing high ratings on the SKAMP to ADHD.

Academic	**Deportment**
#81 _____	#87 _____
#82 _____	#88 _____
#83 _____	#89 _____
#84 _____	#90 _____
#85 _____	
#86 _____	
Total = _____	= _____
Avg. = _____	= _____
Orienting (#81, #86) = _____	Attention to Other (#87, #88) = _____
Maintaining (#82, #83) = _____	Attention to Rules (#89, #90) = _____
Directing (#84, #85) = _____	

Weiss Functional Impairment Scale – Adults 18

18.1 Weiss Functional Impairment Rating Scale (WFIRS) Instructions

Purpose

- ADHD symptoms and actual impairment overlap but are distinct concepts. It is important to measure both since some patients are highly symptomatic but not impaired or vice versa
- This scale contains those items that are most likely to represent the patient's target of treatment. Therefore, the use of the scale before and after treatment can allow the clinician to determine not only if the ADHD has improved, but if the patient's functional difficulties are also better.
- This instrument has been translated into 18 languages. It has been used in many studies and is psychometrically validated. This is the only measure of functional impairment that looks at specific domains and has been validated in the ADHD population.

Design and Validation Information

Scoring The instrument uses a Likert scale such that any item rating 2 or 3 is clinically impaired. The scale can be scored by looking at the total score or by creating a mean score for the total score/number items for each domain, omitting those rated not applicable. For clinical purposes, when defining impairment for DSM-IV, clinicians can consider that any domain with at least two items scored 2, one item scored 3 or a mean score >1.5 is impaired.

Validation The scale has been psychometrically validated with an internal consistency >.8 for each domain and for the scale as a whole. It has moderate convergent validity (0.6) with other measures of functioning (i.e. Columbia Impairment Scale and the Global Assessment of Functioning (GAF)). It has moderate discriminating validity (0.4) from symptoms pre-treatment (i.e. ADHD-Rating Scale) and quality of life (CHIP). The domains have been confirmed by factor analysis, although the domain of school functioning separates into learning and behaviour. The scale is highly sensitive to change with treatment and, in particular, significantly correlated

J. Sadek, *A Clinician's Guide to ADHD*,
DOI 10.1007/978-3-319-02359-5_18, © Springer International Publishing Switzerland 2014

to change in ADHD symptoms (40 % change) and overall psychopathology. Each anchor point on the Likert scale represents approximately one standard deviation (SD). A total score change of 13 would be considered a significant improvement or about half a SD. The change obtained in treatment is typically one full SD. The mean score for risky behaviour in children is 0.5 but increases with age. For adolescents the mean score is 1.

Copyright Information

Margaret D Weiss MD PhD FRCP(C)
Clinic Head, Provincial ADHD Program
Clinical Professor, University of British Columbia
Box 178, 4500 Oak St.
Department of Psychiatry
Children's and Women's Health Centre, Room P-229
Telephone: 604 875 2738 Fax: 604 875 2099
Email: mweiss@cw.bc.ca

Weiss Scale – Parent Reporting

19

J. Sadek, *A Clinician's Guide to ADHD*,
DOI 10.1007/978-3-319-02359-5_19,

CADDRA
CANADIAN ADHD RESOURCE ALLIANCE

Patient Name:
Date of Birth: MRN/File No:
Physician Name: Date:

WEISS FUNCTIONAL IMPAIRMENT RATING SCALE – PARENT REPORT (WFIRS-P)

Your name: ______________________ Relationship to child: ______________

Circle the number for the rating that best describes how your child's emotional or behavioural problems have affected each item in the last month.

		Never or not at all	Sometimes or somewhat	Often or much	Very often or very much	n/a
A	**FAMILY**					
1	Having problems with brothers & sisters	0	1	2	3	n/a
2	Causing problems between parents	0	1	2	3	n/a
3	Takes time away from family members' work or activities	0	1	2	3	n/a
4	Causing fighting in the family	0	1	2	3	n/a
5	Isolating the family from friends and social activities	0	1	2	3	n/a
6	Makes it hard for the family to have fun together	0	1	2	3	n/a
7	Makes parenting difficult	0	1	2	3	n/a
8	Makes it hard to give fair attention to all family members	0	1	2	3	n/a
9	Provokes others to hit or scream at him/her	0	1	2	3	n/a
10	Costs the family more money	0	1	2	3	n/a
B	**SCHOOL**					
	Learning					
1	Makes it difficult to keep up with schoolwork	0	1	2	3	n/a
2	Needs extra help at school	0	1	2	3	n/a
3	Needs tutoring	0	1	2	3	n/a
4	Receives grades that are not as good as his/her ability	0	1	2	3	n/a
	Behaviour					
1	Causes problems for the teacher in the classroom	0	1	2	3	n/a
2	Receives "time-out" or removal from the classroom	0	1	2	3	n/a
3	Having problems in the school yard	0	1	2	3	n/a
4	Receives detentions (during or after school)	0	1	2	3	n/a
5	Suspended or expelled from school	0	1	2	3	n/a
6	Misses classes or is late for school	0	1	2	3	n/a
C	**LIFE SKILLS**					
1	Excessive use of TV, computer, or video games	0	1	2	3	n/a
2	Keeping clean, brushing teeth, brushing hair, bathing, etc.	0	1	2	3	n/a
3	Problems getting ready for school	0	1	2	3	n/a

20 Weiss Scale – Self Report

J. Sadek, *A Clinician's Guide to ADHD*,
DOI 10.1007/978-3-319-02359-5_20, © Springer International Publishing Switzerland 2014

CADDRA
CANADIAN ADHD RESOURCE ALLIANCE

Patient Name:	
Date of Birth:	MRN/File No:
Physician Name:	Date:

WEISS FUNCTIONAL IMPAIRMENT RATING SCALE – SELF REPORT (WFIRS-S)

Name: ______________________________ Date: DD MM YY ________

Date of birth: DD MM YY ________ Sex: ☐ Male ☐ Female
Work: ☐ Full time ☐ Part time ☐ Other ____________
School: ☐ Full time ☐ Part time

Circle the number for the rating that best describes how your emotional or behavioural problems have affected each item in the last month.

		Never or not at all	Sometimes or somewhat	Often or much	Very often or very much	n/a
A	**FAMILY**					
1	Having problems with family	0	1	2	3	n/a
2	Having problems with spouse/partner	0	1	2	3	n/a
3	Relying on others to do things for you	0	1	2	3	n/a
4	Causing fighting in the family	0	1	2	3	n/a
5	Makes it hard for the family to have fun together	0	1	2	3	n/a
6	Problems taking care of your family	0	1	2	3	n/a
7	Problems balancing your needs against those of your family	0	1	2	3	n/
8	Problems losing control with family	0	1	2	3	n/a
B	**WORK**					
1	Problems performing required duties	0	1	2	3	n/a
2	Problems with getting your work done efficiently	0	1	2	3	n/a
3	Problems with your supervisor	0	1	2	3	n/a
4	Problems keeping a job	0	1	2	3	n/a
5	Getting fired from work	0	1	2	3	n/a
6	Problems working in a team	0	1	2	3	n/a
7	Problems with your attendance	0	1	2	3	n/a
8	Problems with being late	0	1	2	3	n/a
9	Problems taking on new tasks	0	1	2	3	n/a
10	Problems working to your potential	0	1	2	3	n/a
11	Poor performance evaluations	0	1	2	3	n/a

Adult ADHD Self-Report Scale (ASRS-v.1.1)

For up-to-date copy of this scale please refer to: http://www.hcp.med.harvard.edu/ncs/asrs.php

Adult ADHD Self-Report Scale (ASRS-v1.1) Symptom Checklist

Patient Name		Today's Date	

Please answer the questions below, rating yourself on each of the criteria shown using the scale on the right side of the page. As you answer each question, place an X in the box that best describes how you have felt and conducted yourself over the past 6 months. Please give this completed checklist to your healthcare professional to discuss during today's appointment.	Never	Rarely	Sometimes	Often	Very Often
1. How often do you have trouble wrapping up the final details of a project, once the challenging parts have been done?					
2. How often do you have difficulty getting things in order when you have to do a task that requires organization?					
3. How often do you have problems remembering appointments or obligations?					
4. When you have a task that requires a lot of thought, how often do you avoid or delay getting started?					
5. How often do you fidget or squirm with your hands or feet when you have to sit down for a long time?					
6. How often do you feel overly active and compelled to do things, like you were driven by a motor?					
					Part A
7. How often do you make careless mistakes when you have to work on a boring or difficult project?					
8. How often do you have difficulty keeping your attention when you are doing boring or repetitive work?					
9. How often do you have difficulty concentrating on what people say to you, even when they are speaking to you directly?					
10. How often do you misplace or have difficulty finding things at home or at work?					
11. How often are you distracted by activity or noise around you?					
12. How often do you leave your seat in meetings or other situations in which you are expected to remain seated?					
13. How often do you feel restless or fidgety?					
14. How often do you have difficulty unwinding and relaxing when you have time to yourself?					
15. How often do you find yourself talking too much when you are in social situations?					
16. When you're in a conversation, how often do you find yourself finishing the sentences of the people you are talking to, before they can finish them themselves?					
17. How often do you have difficulty waiting your turn in situations when turn taking is required?					
18. How often do you interrupt others when they are busy?					
					Part B

20.1 Adult ADHD Self-Report Scale (ASRS v1.1)

20.1.1 Symptoms Checklist Instructions

The questions for the ASRS are designed to stimulate dialogue between you and your patients and to help confirm if they may be suffering from the symptoms of attention-deficit hyperactivity disorder (ADHD).

Description

The Symptom Checklist is an instrument consisting of the 18 DSM-IV-TR criteria. Six of the 18 questions were found to be the most predictive of symptoms consistent with ADHD. These six questions are the basis for the ASRS v1.1 Screener and are also Part A of the Symptom Checklist. Part B of the Symptom Checklist contains the remaining 12 questions.

Instructions

Symptoms

1. Ask the patient to complete both Part A and Part B of the Symptom Checklist by marking an x in the box that most closely represents the frequency of occurrence of each of the symptoms.
2. Score Part A. If four or more marks appear in the darkly shaded boxes within Part A then the patient has symptoms highly consistent with ADHD in adults and further investigation is warranted.
3. The frequency scores on Part B provide additional cues and can serve as further probes into the patient's symptoms. Pay particular attention to marks appearing in the dark shaded boxes. The frequency-based response is more sensitive with certain questions. No total score or diagnostic likelihood is utilized for the 12 questions. It has been found that the six questions in Part A are the most predictive of the disorder and are best for use as a screening instrument.

Impairments

1. Review the entire Symptom Checklist with your patients and evaluate the level of impairment associated with the symptom.
2. Consider work/school, social and family settings.
3. Symptom frequency is often associated with symptom severity, therefore the Symptom Checklist may also aid in the assessment of impairments. If your patients have frequent symptoms, you may want to ask them to describe how these problems have affected the ability to work, take care of things at home, or get along with other people such as their spouse/significant other.

History

1. Assess the presence of these symptoms or similar symptoms in childhood. Adults who have ADHD need not have been formally diagnosed on childhood. In evaluating a patient's history, look for evidence of early-appearing and long-standing problems with attention or self-control. Some significant symptoms should have been present in childhood, but fully symptomology is not necessary.

The value of screening for Adults with ADHD

Research suggests that the symptoms of ADHD can persist into adulthood, having a significant impact on relationships, careers, and even the personal safety of your patients who may suffer from it (Schweitzer et al. 2001; Barkley 2005; Biederman et al. 1993; American psychiatric Association 2000). Because this disorder is often misunderstood, many people who have it do not receive appropriate treatment and, as a result, may never reach their full potential. Part of the problem is that it can be difficult to diagnose, particularly in adults.

The Adult ADHD Self-Report Scale (ASRS-v1.1) Symptom Checklist was developed in conjunction with the World Health Organization (WHO), and the Workgroup on Adult ADHD that included the following team of psychiatrists and researchers:

- Lenard Adler, MD, Associate Professor of Psychiatry and Neurology
- Ronald C. Kessler, PhD, Professor, Department of Health Care Policy, Harvard Medical School
- Thomas Spencer, MD, Associate Professor of Psychiatry, Harvard Medical School

As the healthcare professional, you can use the ASRS v1.1 as a tool to help screen for ADHD in adult patients. Insights gained through this screening may suggest the need for a more in-depth clinician review. The questions in the ASRS v1.1 are consistent with DSM-IV criteria and address the manifestations of ADHD symptoms in adults. Content of the questionnaire also reflects the importance that DSM-IV places on symptoms, impairments, and history for a correct diagnosis (American Psychiatric Association 2000).

The checklist takes about minutes to complete and can provide information that is critical to supplement the diagnostic process.

For up-to-date copy of this scale please refer to: http://www.hcp.med.harvard.edu/ncs/asrs.php

References

American Psychiatric Association (2000) Diagnostic manual of mental disorders, 4th edn, text revision. American Psychiatric Association, Washington, DC, pp 85–93

Barkley RA (2005) Attention deficit hyperactivity disorder: a handbook for diagnostic and treatment, 2nd edn. Guilford Press, New York

Biederman J et al (1993) Patterns of psychiatric comorbidity, cognition, and psychosocial functioning in adults with attention deficit hyperactivity disorder. Am J Psychiatry 150:1792–1798

Schweitzer JB et al (2001) Attention deficit hyperactivity disorder Med Clin N Am 85(3):10–11, 757–777

Sadek Personal Adversity Questionnaire – Adults

21

21.1 Sadek Personal Adversity Questionnaire (S-PAQ)©

Permission to reproduce may be obtained from Dr. Joseph Sadek email: joseph.sadek@cdha.nshealth.ca

This scale is designed for the patient to complete and designed for adults to help in the diagnosing for ADHD.

Please circle the answer that applies to you.			
1. My mom's pregnancy was complicated by her smoking or her use of street drugs or alcohol.	*True*	*False*	*Unsure*
2. My birth was difficulty and complicated.	*True*	*False*	*Unsure*
3. I was delayed in talking or walking.	*True*	*False*	*Unsure*
4. I has problems with becoming toilet trained.	*True*	*False*	*Unsure*
5. I was bullied as a child.	*True*	*False*	*Unsure*
6. I was sexually abused between ages 5–10.	*True*	*False*	*Unsure*
7. I was sexually abused between ages 11–15.	*True*	*False*	*Unsure*
8. I was physically abused.	*True*	*False*	*Unsure*
9. I failed one grade at school.	*True*	*False*	*Unsure*
10. I failed more than one grade at school.	*True*	*False*	*Unsure*
11. I had serious academic difficulties in school. I went for special education or resource classes.	*True*	*False*	*Unsure*
12. Teachers did not like me.	*True*	*False*	*Unsure*
13. I had very few friends in school.	*True*	*False*	*Unsure*
14. I was a shy and timid child.	*True*	*False*	*Unsure*
15. I did not get along well with my siblings.	*True*	*False*	*Unsure*
16. I grew up in a poor family.	*True*	*False*	*Unsure*
17. I always felt inferior to others.	*True*	*False*	*Unsure*
18. I was ashamed of who I was as a child.	*True*	*False*	*Unsure*
19. It was difficult to separate from my parents.	*True*	*False*	*Unsure*
20. I hated going to school.	*True*	*False*	*Unsure*
21. School was a source of stress for me.	*True*	*False*	*Unsure*
22. As a teenager, I felt like a failure.	*True*	*False*	*Unsure*

(continued)

J. Sadek, *A Clinician's Guide to ADHD*,
DOI 10.1007/978-3-319-02359-5_21, © Springer International Publishing Switzerland 2014

23. My mother was not affectionate with me, and/or did not show her caring for me.	*True*	*False*	*Unsure*
24. My father was not affectionate with me, and/or did not show his caring for me.	*True*	*False*	*Unsure*
25. My parents were not well off and my needs were not met as a child.	*True*	*False*	*Unsure*
26. My parents separated when I was less than 10 years old.	*True*	*False*	*Unsure*
27. My parents separated when I was less than 20 years old.	*True*	*False*	*Unsure*
28. My parents were authoritarians and controlling.	*True*	*False*	*Unsure*
29. I had difficulty paying attention at home and at school.	*True*	*False*	*Unsure*
30. I was a hyperactive child. I couldn't sit still.	*True*	*False*	*Unsure*
31. I am always on the go.	*True*	*False*	*Unsure*
32. People say I talk too much.	*True*	*False*	*Unsure*
33. I'm loud and people notice that.	*True*	*False*	*Unsure*
34. I feel restless every day.	*True*	*False*	*Unsure*
35. I leave my seat during meetings because I cannot sit for a long time.	*True*	*False*	*Unsure*
36. I can't relax.	*True*	*False*	*Unsure*
37. My room/car is usually a mess.	*True*	*False*	*Unsure*
38. I can't keep focusing for more than 10 min on topics that I don't like.	*True*	*False*	*Unsure*
39. I often misplace things like my keys, wallet, glasses, and use to lose things as a child.	*True*	*False*	*Unsure*
40. I can start projects but not finish them.	*True*	*False*	*Unsure*
41. I am distractible	*True*	*False*	*Unsure*
42. My memory is poor. I need reminders and organizers.	*True*	*False*	*Unsure*
43. I have trouble noticing details.	*True*	*False*	*Unsure*
44. I am told I am a bad listener.	*True*	*False*	*Unsure*
45. I drive impulsively.	*True*	*False*	*Unsure*
46. I was an impulsive child, could not wait my turn, I blurt out answers and interrupted others.	*True*	*False*	*Unsure*
47. I set fires on purpose as a child.	*True*	*False*	*Unsure*
48. I was charged many times.	*True*	*False*	*Unsure*
49. I stole before the age of 10 many times.	*True*	*False*	*Unsure*
50. I stole after the age of 10 many times.	*True*	*False*	*Unsure*
51. I started many physical fights.	*True*	*False*	*Unsure*
52. I bullied other kids.	*True*	*False*	*Unsure*
53. I started drinking as a teenager.	*True*	*False*	*Unsure*
54. I started using street drugs as a teenager.	*True*	*False*	*Unsure*
55. As a teenager, I was arrested more than once.	*True*	*False*	*Unsure*
56. I was a defiant and spiteful child.	*True*	*False*	*Unsure*
57. I did not respect authorities.	*True*	*False*	*Unsure*

If patients answers with several true responses to questions 29–46 then further inquiry into ADHD is needed.

Questions 47–55 point to further inquiry into conduct disorder.

Questions 56–58 point to ODD further inquiry.

Sadek Personality Difficulties Questionnaire – Adults

22

22.1 Sadek Personality Difficulties Questionnaire (S-PDQ)©

Permission to reproduce may be obtained from Dr. Joseph Sadek email: joseph.sadek@cdha.nshealth.ca

This scale is designed for the patient to complete and designed for adults to help in the diagnosing for issues **other than** ADHD.

Please circle the answer that applies to you.			
1. I never keep a job for more than 6 months.	*True*	*False*	*Unsure*
2. I never felt competent at my work.	*True*	*False*	*Unsure*
3. I never enjoyed my work.	*True*	*False*	*Unsure*
4. I have problems with my identity.	*True*	*False*	*Unsure*
5. I had sexual encounters with the same sex.	*True*	*False*	*Unsure*
6. My intimate relationships never last for more than 6 months.	*True*	*False*	*Unsure*
7. I had too many sexual partners to count.	*True*	*False*	*Unsure*
8. I cannot keep friends.	*True*	*False*	*Unsure*
9. My emotions are like a roller coaster, shifting quickly.	*True*	*False*	*Unsure*
10. I feel empty most of the time.	*True*	*False*	*Unsure*
11. For years li have had regular suicidal thoughts/behavior.	*True*	*False*	*Unsure*
12. I feel like killing myself if I am abandoned.	*True*	*False*	*Unsure*
13. I cannot control my anger most of the time.	*True*	*False*	*Unsure*
14. I feel special and unique with lots of talents.	*True*	*False*	*Unsure*
15. People are there to serve me.	*True*	*False*	*Unsure*
16. I think that most people are ignorant and stupid.	*True*	*False*	*Unsure*
17. People bring the misery on themselves/they deserve it.	*True*	*False*	*Unsure*
18. My friends are in high places.	*True*	*False*	*Unsure*
19. I do not care about the law, I have my own laws.	*True*	*False*	*Unsure*
20. I drive recklessly.	*True*	*False*	*Unsure*
21. I lie to get what I want.	*True*	*False*	*Unsure*
22. I do not plan ahead.	*True*	*False*	*Unsure*
23. I do not think people are loyal to anyone.	*True*	*False*	*Unsure*
24. I do not forgive insults.	*True*	*False*	*Unsure*
25. I cannot confide in anyone.	*True*	*False*	*Unsure*

(continued)

J. Sadek, *A Clinician's Guide to ADHD*,
DOI 10.1007/978-3-319-02359-5_22, © Springer International Publishing Switzerland 2014

26. I do not trust people.	*True*	*False*	*Unsure*
27. I cannot get involved with people unless I am liked.	*True*	*False*	*Unsure*
28. I worry a lot about people criticizing me.	*True*	*False*	*Unsure*
29. I avoid social situations most of the time.	*True*	*False*	*Unsure*
30. I cannot make decisions without lots of advice from others.	*True*	*False*	*Unsure*
31. I would do anything to get approval from others.	*True*	*False*	*Unsure*

Questions 1–13 points to Borderline Personality disorder
Questions 14–18 points to Narcissistic Personality Disorder
Questions 19–22 points to Antisocial Personality disorder
Questions 23–26 points to paranoid personality disorder
Questions 27–31 points to dependant avoidant personality traits

22.2 Diagnostic Interview for ADHD in Adults (DIVA)

The **DIVA** is based on the DSM-IV criteria and is the first structured Dutch interview for ADHD in adults. The DIVA has been developed by J.J.S. Kooji and M.H. Francken and is the successor of the earlier Semi-Structured Interview for ADHD in adults (Kooji 2010; Kooji and Francken 2007).

In order to simplify the evaluation of each of the 18 symptom criteria for ADHD, in childhood and adulthood, the interview provides a list of concrete and realistic examples, for both current and retrospective (childhood) behavior. The examples are also provided of the types of impairments that are commonly associated with the symptoms in five areas of everyday life: work and education; relationships and family life; social contacts; free time and hobbies; self-confidence and self-image.

Wherever possible the DIVA should be completed with adults in the presence of a partner and/or family member, to enable retrospective and collateral information to be ascertained at the same time. The DIVA usually takes around one and a half hours to complete.

The DIVA only asks about the core symptoms of ADHD required to make the DSM-IV diagnosis of ADHD, and does not ask about other co-occurring psychiatric symptoms, syndromes or disorders. However comorbidity is commonly seen in both children and adults in ADHD, in around 75 % of cases. For this reason, it is important to complete a general psychiatric assessment to enquire about commonly co-occurring symptoms, syndromes and disorders. The most common mental health problems that accompany ADHD include anxiety, depression, bipolar disorder, substance abuse disorders and addiction, sleep problems and personality disorders, and all these should be investigated. This is needed to understand the full range of symptoms experienced by the individual with ADHD; and also for the differential diagnosis, to exclude other major psychiatric disorders as the primary cause of 'ADHD symptoms' in adults (Kooji and Francken 2007).

The Diagnostic Interview for ADHD in adults (DIVA) is a publication of the DIVA Foundation, The Hague, The Netherlands, August, 2010. Reprinted with permission form the Diagnostic Statistical Manual of Mental Disorders, Text Revision, Fourth Edition (Copyright 2000). American Psychiatric Association.

To view the most current version please, refer to www.divacenter.eu.

References

Diagnostic Interview for ADHD in Adults 2.0 (DIVA2.0) (2010) In: Kooji JJS. Adult ADHD. Diagnostic assessment and treatment. Pearson Assessment and Information BV, Amsterdam

Kooji JJS, Francken MH (2007) Diagnostich Interview Voor ADHD (DIVA) bij volwassenen. Online available at www.kenniscentrumadhdbijvolwassenen.nl, 2007 and published in English in reference 2

Websites

ADHD Guidelines Available on the Internet

Canadian ADHD Guidelines: http://www.caddra.ca/cms4/

American Psychological Association: http://www.apa.org/topics/adhd/index.aspx

Scottish ADHD Guidelines: http://www.sign.ac.uk/guidelines/fulltext/112/index.html

National Institute for Health and Clinical Excellence NICE http://publications.nice.org.uk/attention-deficit-hyperactivity-disorder-cg72

Australian ADHD Draft Guidelines: http://www.nhmrc.gov.au/guidelines/publications/ch54

Other Websites of Interest

A. ADDitude: Living well with Attention Deficit Magazine http://www.additudemag.com
B. ADDvance: Answers to Your Questions about ADD (ADHD) http://www.addvance.com
C. American Academy of Child and Adolescent Psychiatry (AACAP) http://www.aacap.org
D. American Academy of Family Physicians (AAFP) http://www.aafp.org/online/en/home.html
E. American Academy of Pediatrics (AAP) http://www.aap.org and http://www.healthychildren.org
F. American Association of People with Disabilities (AAPD) http://www.aapd.com
G. American Medical Association (AMA) http://www.ama-assn.org
H. Attention Deficit Disorder Association (ADDA) http://www.add.org
I. CADDRA http://www.caddra.ca
J. Centre for Disease Control http://www.cdc.gov/ncbddd/actearly/pdf/parents_pdfs/adhdfactsheet.pdf
K. Children and Adults with Attention Deficit/Hyperactivity Disorder (HADD) http://www.chadd.org
L. Consortium for Citizens with Disabilities (CCD) http://www.c-c-d.org/
M. Council for Learning Disabilities (CLD) http://www.cldinternational.org/
N. Internet Mental Health http://www.mentalhealth.com/
O. Learning Disabilities Association of America (LDA) http://www.ldanatl.org/

J. Sadek, *A Clinician's Guide to ADHD*,
DOI 10.1007/978-3-319-02359-5,

P. Lives in the Balance http://www.livesinthebalance.org/
Q. National Dissemination Center for Children with Disabilities (NICHCY) http://nichcy.org/
R. National Alliance on Mental Illness http://www.nami.org/
S. National Clearing House http://www.help4adhd.org/
T. National Institute of Mental Health (NIMH) http://www.nimh.nih.gov/health/topics/attention-deficit-hyperactivity-disorder-adhd/index.shtml
U. Northern County Psychiatric Association http://www.ncpamd.com/
V. Parent Advocacy Coalition for Educational Rights (PACER) Center http://www.pacer.org/
W. Substance Abuse & Mental Health Services Administration (SAMHSA) http://www.samhsa.gov/

Canadian publishing number ISBN – 978-0-9881243-0-1

The manufacturer's authorised representative in the EU is Springer Nature Customer Service Centre GmbH, Europaplatz 3, 69115 Heidelberg, Germany. If you have any concerns regarding our products, please contact ProductSafety@springernature.com

Printed and bound by CPI Group (UK) Ltd, Croydon, CR0 4YY
30/09/2026
02225578-0003